The
Bedroom
Gap

The
Bedroom
Gap

Rewrite the Rules and Roles
of Sex in Midlife

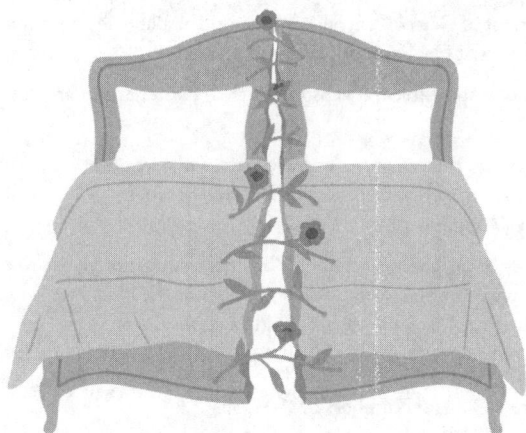

Maria Sophocles, MD

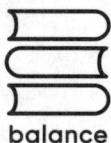

balance

New York   Boston

Balance
Hachette Book Group
1290 Avenue of the Americas
New York, NY 10104
GCP-Balance.com
@GCPBalance

First Edition: February 2026

Balance is an imprint of Grand Central Publishing. The Balance name and logo are registered trademarks of Hachette Book Group, Inc.

The publisher is not responsible for websites (or their content) that are not owned by the publisher.

The Hachette Speakers Bureau provides a wide range of authors for speaking events. To find out more, go to hachettespeakersbureau.com or email HachetteSpeakers@hbgusa.com.

Balance books may be purchased in bulk for business, educational, or promotional use. For information, please contact your local bookseller or the Hachette Book Group Special Markets Department at special.markets@hbgusa.com.

Print book interior design by Bart Dawson.

Library of Congress Control Number: 2025035553

ISBNs: 9780306837401 (hardcover), 9780306837425 (ebook)

Printed in the United States of America

LSC-C

Printing 1, 2025

For Bear:
"I was born to join in love, not hate."
—Sophocles (*Antigone*)

For Alex and Em:
"The loyal heart is a quiet force—it endures,
even when unrecognized."—Anonymous

For Thomas:
"A sensitive heart absorbs beauty others walk past."
—Bob the Fat Tomato

For Christian:
"Energy and persistence conquer all things."
—Benjamin Franklin

For Katerina Eleni:
"If you suddenly and unexpectedly feel joy, don't hesitate.
Give in to it . . . whatever it is, don't be afraid of its plenty.
Joy is not made to be a crumb."—Mary Oliver

For George and Annette Sophocles:
"One word frees us of all the weight and pain of life:
That word is love."—Sophocles

Contents

"Women's degradation is in man's idea of his sexual rights. Our religion, laws, customs, are all founded on the belief that woman was made for man."

—Elizabeth Cady Stanton

Introduction

One of my patients, a member of the Screen Actors Guild, had invited me to the premier of *On the Basis of Sex*, the movie about Ruth Bader Ginsburg's early years. After the screening, RBG herself took the stage as NPR's Nina Totenberg interviewed her. I was seated in the third row; just behind me to my right was Hilary Clinton and to her left was Gloria Steinem. Seated at the vertex of these feminist icons, I felt inspired just being there. But it was at the after-party that the empowerment factor really amped up.

While other guests of honor departed after RBG's interview, Gloria Steinem stuck around. She was surrounded by selfie-seeking fans and women wanting to tell her about a march or a conference they had attended, hoping to get a smile and some encouragement from the feminist goddess. In all honesty, I didn't want to bother her, but a little bit later, when I went to retrieve my coat, I found her in the cloak room, alone. I did the awkward greeting-acknowledgment-approval nod and, to my surprise, she would have none of it.

"Who are you, and what's your story?" she asked. I shared, of course, and we began an easy and natural conversation. She was, as if in a movie about herself, fiery, passionate, determined, and not a whit jaded or tired. She was as engaging, captivating, and motivating as one would expect her to be. Four-letter invectives about misogynist politicians whirred around that coatroom as we shared condemnation and concern about the "state of affairs" with respect to women's rights in general. Then we went on at length about the blatant gender bias in biomedical research, in clinical medicine, in reproductive rights . . . and in the bedroom.

"How the hell are we supposed to get consensus, to make progress, when our own f—ing president is grabbing pussies?" she complained.

"Well why not?" I countered cheekily, seeing her eyebrows raise, "when women don't expect to be treated equally in their own bedrooms? When we play these stupid submissive sex roles because our mothers or grandmothers or television taught us that sex is for men, that pleasure is for men? Why wouldn't a powerful man—or any man—assume sex is his for the taking, that he is *entitled* to it?" Her ire was up, and so was mine. Yup, this patriarchal bullshit was not just political, it was happening right in our bedrooms. And it was pervasive.

"You better write that damn book," Steinem told me. "Write it now. Write like your house is on fire. Write like women's lives depend on it, Maria. Because they do."

My mission was clear. Gloria Steinem herself had commanded it. But as I drove to my clinic to see patients the following day, I felt the full weight of the task ahead of me. Which is to say, I felt the weight of several huge forces—history, patriarchy, educational want, medical aloofness, and media misinformation—that have created and perpetuated unequal, gendered roles in the bedroom. I refer to this phenomenon as the Bedroom Gap. It involves the difference between what men and women think, expect, and experience sexually, and it is deeply embedded into our society.

As an ob/gyn focusing on menopause, I am interested in a specific aspect of the Bedroom Gap: It only gets wider as we age. Why is that? It is because there is a maddeningly huge, self-esteem damaging, relationship-wrecking gap between the discourse about sexual issues related to menopause and what's happening behind closed doors. The public discrepancy, in which the medical community ignores or glosses over what women are going through during this life phase, and the private one, a gendered, intensely personal gap playing out in bedrooms all over the world, are deeply connected. The two Bedroom Gaps reinforce each other, intertwined like the double helix of a socio-sexual DNA.

If you're reading this and thinking, "But celebrities talk about menopause all the time! Oprah has a whole curriculum on it," you're not wrong. It's not *whether* they're talking about it, but *how* they're talking about it. Yes, we are, as a society, finally talking about *menopause* in public, thanks in no small part to the demographic explosion of menopausal women and the burgeoning multibillion dollar women's health–focused tech sector. But what is being said about *sex in menopause* remains scant, weak, and insignificant, like a middling orgasm during which you're still thinking about the soup on the stove or your kid's failing calculus grade.

Let's do a little compare and contrast exercise. Here are three high-profile women talking menopause.

Gwyneth Paltrow has been quoted saying, "I think when you get into perimenopause, you notice a lot of changes. I can feel the hormonal changes happening, the sweating, the moods—you know you're just, like, all of a sudden furious for no reason."

Michelle Obama has shared, "It was like somebody put a furnace in my core and turned it on high, and then everything started melting. And I thought, 'Well, this is crazy. I can't, I can't, I can't do this.'"

And then we have this description from *Sex in the City*'s Kim Catrall: "Literally one moment you're fine, and then another, you feel like you're in a vat of boiling water, and you feel like the rug has been pulled out from underneath you."

Hot flashes: Check. Mood changes: Check. Out-of-body experience: Check. I know the power of a celebrity endorsement, and so while I applaud their semitransparency, I call bullshit on these paparazzi peeks into Menopause Experiences of the Rich and Famous. If you've experienced menopause, you know full well that celebrities aren't telling the whole story. They are giving us snippets we can relate to while keeping their red carpet glam and their marketability as strong sexy women (with flawless skin and full-bodied hair) intact. Until recently—thank you, Halle Berry and Naomi Watts—there was an utter lack of admission that there are any vaginal or sexual issues going on during this life phase.

Now for the compare and contrast part. Here's a sample of what my menopausal patients tell me:

- "I think my vagina is broken or something."
- "My vagina has betrayed me."
- "My vagina no longer listens to me; she's a naughty girl."
- "My vagina feels drier than the Sahara. Like the walls are sandpaper."
- "It feels like shards of glass in there when I have sex."
- "It feels like tissue paper, it feels like it tears and splits when he's in there."
- "I bleed when we have sex and it is so embarrassing and it ruins the mood for him."
- "I couldn't care less if I ever had sex again. My libido is less than zero."

Celebrities are willing to share how embarrassing it is to be sweaty and grouchy, but they aren't willing to say that they're suffering from lack of libido, sexual pain, or an inability to orgasm. After all, what would Hollywood be without the illusion of sexual vibrancy and eternal youth?

But it's not just celebrities. So few women in this life phase are willing to really discuss the nitty gritty sexual details of what they are experiencing. This misplaced sense of shame and the resulting lack of open, honest conversations about the full range of symptoms of menopause does a grave disservice to all of us. We end up thinking that if we are experiencing *sexual* versions of menopause mayhem, there must be something wrong with us, even as we start to talk openly about the myriad symptoms of menopause that have nothing to do with what's going on in our bedrooms.

It used to be unacceptable to talk about depression, or about one's sexual preferences, or about gender identity. These topics have had their coming out, and while resistance remains in some conservative communities—and the resulting political feeding frenzies are excellent clickbait—societies are better for it. As I write this, menopause itself is coming out of the closet—it's about time!—but the *sexual fallout* from menopause remains a mostly untold story. I am counting the days until a public discussion of menopause-related sexual issues is as acceptable as crying during an Oscars acceptance speech.

If you picked up this book, I'm guessing you have unanswered questions resulting from your own sexual journey. Maybe your menopausal changes are bringing this issue to an uncomfortable level of awareness. Maybe you've mentioned sexual symptoms to your doctor and they deflected or demurred or even ignored you. I apologize if you were ever dismissed or made to feel insignificant by a clinician. I also salute your doctor if they earnestly listen and give patients an empathetic ear, despite what is likely to be minimal training in sexual medicine.

Maybe you haven't found the words, or a sympathetic ear, or a helpful resource that gives you some space to talk about what's happening to you sexually right now. Maybe you feel at your age and stage that it doesn't matter or that there is nothing you can do about it. I want you to know that whether you are menopausal or not, *it matters if you have unresolved issues in your sex life*, and this book is for you.

Education Deficit

The menopausal Bedroom Gap refers to all the differences you are experiencing in your sex life at this age. These include differences in sexual expectations, in sexual performance, even just in thoughts about how we're supposed to behave in a sexually intimate setting. While some of you who are reading this book are heterosexual couples without major health issues, Bedroom Gaps exist in all kinds of bedrooms—affecting gay couples, disabled couples, women who are cancer survivors, assault and childhood abuse survivors, victims of genital mutilation, and other under-the-radar groups. Bedroom Gaps are also common among women raised in conservative communities or households that did not mention sex and valued chastity.

If we think of Bedroom Gaps as a reflection of education—and I don't mean the school kind—the discrepancies are widest at the beginning and end of our reproductive lifespans, two life chapters packed with changes and uncertainty, where education, information, and the assurance that you are normal is imperative. This is when we most need to understand our bodies, our sexual selves, and those of our partners. While my thoughts on the sexual messages and (mis)education of adolescents and young adults could fill a whole book, most of this book will focus on the sexual issues of midlife and later.

Options Lacking

Whoopi Goldberg described the Bedroom Gap perfectly during a standup routine many years ago: "How can you keep a man [erect] for 19 hours and not be able to cool down a hot flash?" She was referring to Viagra, which has done a remarkable job widening the Bedroom Gap between men and women by increasing the sexual performance discrepancy. Thankfully we are making inroads into hot flashes; in 2023, the FDA approved the first nonhormonal medication for hot flashes. But even the fearless Whoopi didn't go as far as to mention that we don't really have a Viagra counterpart for women. In Chapter 2, we'll get into the reasons why the Little Pink Pill for women didn't pack the ejaculatory punch that the Little Blue Pill did for men, and why it didn't turn out to be profitable for Big Pharma to pursue.

Vaginal Estrogen:
An Untapped Fountain of Youth

It's not that there aren't prescription options to help women with sexual issues. Topical estrogen was the first product developed and marketed to improve the vagina's integrity. It launched in 1946, it's still on the market today, and it works. It is safe and effective liquid gold. But this antiaging elixir remains largely untapped. Why? At least two reasons. First, estrogen has a reputation problem, thanks to twenty-year-old, outdated, and disproven studies suggesting increased cancer risk that resulted in a widespread fear among women and clinicians that persists today. Second, the FDA has a nasty little habit called class labeling, which has misled and struck unnecessary fear into label-reading women everywhere. More on both later in this book—because the pharmaceutical industry is on my list of things we absolutely need to talk about when we address menopause and sex.

The Research Gap

Whoopi's comment cited earlier highlights the tremendous gap in medical research and development related to men and women. The fact that we have had so few pharmaceutical options for women's menopausal and sexual health, as well as the fact that so many studies have actually used men rather than women as subjects, underscores the need for a top-down restructuring of the research industry. Women are in fact *not* just small versions of men. We are our own gender of the human species, and we merit studies and R&D and investment funding as much as men. Menopause, the sleeping giant, the life chapter that affects 100 percent of women, is finally waking, but the sexual issues it causes could use attention. As progressive a society as America seems, it remains mired in prudishness, stuck in age-old sex role stereotypes that dictate it is not polite or normal for women to discuss or complain about sex.

Try as we might to sweep it under the rug, there is a clear difference in what happens in a bedroom between men and women in middle age. That gap is widened and made worse by a lack of knowledge about what happens to women's bodies in midlife.

Here's my promise to you: We're going to get brutally honest about what is actually happening at this stage of your life. It's high time the nearly eighty million currently menopausal women in the United States alone get the tools they need to actually do something about their own Bedroom Gap.

And yes, I said eighty million. As I write this in 2025, nearly all the female baby boomers (born between 1946 and 1964) and plenty of Generation X women (born between 1965 and 1980) are menopausal. That adds up to eighty million menopausal women right now in the United States and close to a billion worldwide. An additional six thousand women in America hit menopause every single day.

We're talking about a lot of women being left high and (sometimes painfully) dry.

Why is this population largely ignored? Because *how we approach sex in midlife reflects not just misinformation but an androcentric model of sex that's been in place for more than four thousand years.*

A History Lesson

Let's take a whirlwind historical sex tour and enumerate just a few highlights to see what I mean:

Hysterical Virgins

In Ancient Greece, the city of Argos had a serious problem: A group of virgins was refusing to "honor the phallus." Behaving strangely and hallucinating, these women refused to have sex and fled to the mountains. The ruler of Argos asked Melampus, a local physician and perhaps the founder of psychiatry, to help solve this bizarre situation. Melampus urged the women to have sex to clear their heads and to resolve what he determined to be symptoms of hysteria (from the Greek word for uterus). He attributed their madness to a poisoned uterus brought on by a lack of orgasms and uterine melancholy. This diagnosis stemmed from the idea that sexual inactivity was not a great thing and that men needed to have sex with women to purge the latter's uteri of the toxins that would build up if the women did not have sex. Hmmm. What a convenient diagnosis.

Vulva Shaming

Anatomist Andreas Vesalius (born 1514) named the external genitalia Pudendum, from the Latin "to make ashamed." Enough said on that one, don't you think? I have seen a thousand penises glorified in marble, but the vulva has never really gotten its due. It is usually portrayed as just a shameful little wedge of skin and hair instead of the unique and beautiful flowerlike object it is.

The Treatment of Desire

Then there was Victorian-era hysteria, which saw nineteenth-century male MDs trying to explain and "treat" female desire. Even though the veracity of the well-known stereotype of male clinicians masturbating their female patients to "cure" hysteria has been debated, much of our present day sexual misunderstanding about female desire and orgasm can be traced to Sigmund Freud.[1] More on this later.

Clitoris Confusion

Marie Bonaparte, Napoleon's great-grandniece, was so unsatisfied sexually that she studied and blamed the location of a woman's clitoris for lack of orgasm. She hypothesized that the farther the clitoris from the vaginal opening, the less likely a woman was to orgasm. Never mind the contribution—or lack thereof—from inept sexual partners, her theory was that it all came down to the anatomy you were born with. She believed so vehemently in her theory, even publishing a medical paper on the subject under a male pseudonym, that she underwent two surgical procedures (since the first yielded no sexual satisfaction) to move her clitoris closer to the vaginal opening. (This confusion over clitorises, sadly, hasn't changed much—it wasn't until 2005, when the full anatomy of the clitoris was revealed, that the clitoris was accurately represented in medical textbooks.)

Why do I share this history? Because I believe that learning about beliefs and cultural patterns from the past helps us understand our present and improve our future. It also helps us feel less like this is "only my problem" when, in fact, the way we feel about female sexual concepts—desire, pleasure, performance—can be traced back through centuries of embedded beliefs.

Indeed, that millennia-old androcentric sex model is (still) impacting our physical and mental health, our self-esteem, and our relationships. It's hard to change pesky little habits we've all picked up over the years, let alone undo four thousand years of women not being asked what they need in bed, not to mention never finding societal permission to ask.

Another reason we're behind on addressing female sexual pleasure relates to changing lifespans. Before the twentieth century, women in industrialized countries could expect to live to sixty years old, barely a decade after menopause. Women's post-reproductive years were focused on home duties and their sexuality in this life stage was never spoken of. Sex was for procreation, and women's sexual pleasure was simply not on anyone's radar and, if it was, was treated as a scandalous topic. Meanwhile, sex for men has always been both procreative and pleasurable, through the ages and at all ages. You see the magnitude of the discrepancy?

Today, women live more than a third of their lives after menopause. Yet we don't treat their experiences much differently than we did 120-plus years ago.

A Med Ed Gap

Ironically, one of places you won't find helpful information on the menopausal years is in medical education, which remains stubbornly resistant to addressing female-only conditions, including menopause, and adopting a progressive model of sexual health. Even today, only a small fraction of ob/gyns are trained in menopause, even though 100 percent of their Assigned Female at Birth (AFAB) patients will become menopausal. Furthermore, even though menopause affects pretty much every organ, tissue, and cell in a woman's body, only 7 percent of ob/gyn residents felt comfortable managing menopause by the end of their training.

I was part of the menopause and sexual health–uninformed clinical corps. After eight years of training to become an ob/gyn—four in medical school and another four in residency—I still had no clue about menopause or sexual dysfunction. And I definitely had no clue how much the former affected the latter.

After my residency, I joined a private practice in a tony suburb of Philadelphia, confident in my training. After all, I was adept at delivering babies. I could perform complex laparoscopic surgeries. I'd studied with nationally known ob/gyns from Johns Hopkins. I felt prepared. Cocky, even.

My pregnant twenty- and thirtysomething patients were a breeze. I could counsel them about pregnancy without a moment's hesitation. Then, I found myself face-to-face with a woman in her mid-fifties. She quietly apologized for feeling "off." When I asked her to explain, she elaborated, "I'm quick to tears and quick to snap at my husband and I feel stupid around my coworkers because I can't recall words sometimes." She continued, "I have joint aches and feel tired all the time. I wake up during the night and have trouble getting back to sleep. I have no sexual interest at all. If I never had sex again, that would be fine with me."

This woman felt like a mess. And I had no idea what to tell her. Her symptoms were so varied and all over the map, I couldn't figure out whether she needed a neurologist, a gastroenterologist, a rheumatologist, or a psychiatrist. Nothing made sense; nothing coincided with any particular organ system or specialty. Perplexed and even skeptical (did she have a drug dependency?), I decided I wasn't qualified to help her and dutifully gave her the names of local internists and psychotherapists. Then I left the room. In retrospect, I pretty much walked out on her, unaware that I was her last big hope.

I couldn't have done a worse job. And while that was 1995, even today clinicians everywhere couldn't be doing a worse job. They are failing their patients, and most of them don't even know it because their medical school education failed *them*. A 2019 study showed that 20.3 percent of residents in ob/gyn, family medicine, and internal medicine received no training at all in menopause. So it comes as little surprise that only 6.8 percent of residents reported feeling adequately prepared to treat menopausal patients.

It gets worse. Being "trained in menopause" basically means your medical school devoted more than five minutes to teaching the topic. It probably means the professors focused on the physiology part (in short, this is the life period where the ovaries stop making hormones) and not what happens clinically (and in real life) to women as a *result* of these changes. In residency, there's little to no training on how to care for patients with menopause in a comprehensive way. No focus on alternative and nonmedical therapies, hormonal and nonhormonal therapies. No commitment to helping future doctors understand the myriad presentations of menopausal issues, from palpitations to hair loss to joint pain. And definitely no focus on sexual dysfunction.

But wait, there's more. Even clinicians with menopause training often don't feel personally comfortable talking about menopausal issues. We will read in Chapter 7 how most of the senior residents on the brink of finishing all that training say they do not feel comfortable talking about menopause treatments.[2] Many bring their own discomfort into the exam room. They prejudge women as "lazy" or "complainers" and prioritize avoidance over helpfulness. When I interviewed for jobs just fifteen years ago, many ob/gyns I spoke with told me they just hoped the menopausal patients wouldn't "open their mouths," or that I should "just hope they don't wreck your schedule with all the stuff in their head." My colleague Dr. Somi Javaid shared that an ob/gyn once told her, "I can't even get my wife interested in sex, how am I supposed to know how to help my patients with sex?"

It's not just doctors who aren't getting the education we deserve—the general population isn't, either. Whether or not you had decent sex ed classes growing up, you likely also grew up with plenty of lessons about sex from pop culture. If you aren't really sure if what I'm telling you is true, that sexual power and sexual decision-making has always been in the hands and bodies of men, look no further than the Disney princesses.

(If you're a die-hard Disney fan and don't want to risk me ruining the classics for you, I suggest you skip this part.)

Snow White, released in 1937, has not aged well in terms of bedroom politics. She is basically either dead or comatose from biting a poisoned apple, and the only "cure" is a kiss by the prince; no need to value her mind, her character, her wit, or her education, and no need for her to have an opinion or a voice for that matter. Consent? Nope. Oh and by the way, she's *fourteen*! *Cinderella* (1950) features a (beautiful, slim, blonde) woman stuck in domestic servitude until she is discovered at a ball; her looks alone (and a tiny dainty foot that can slip into a delicate glass slipper) somehow win the heart of the prince, who pursues her and gives her a life of riches in return for being his arm candy. Sadly, we, the viewers, know she is in fact kind and caring, but these qualities are swept under the rug and not valued by either the prince or the film's director. Even as late as 1989, Disney's *Little Mermaid* was unabashedly reinforcing the narrative that women who relinquish their agency—sexual, intellectual, even vocal—are preferable to men. Ursula the "Sea Witch" advises Ariel that men on land don't care for women who "blabber."

My patients grew up in an era when the princesses they idolized married princes who valued their looks, took care of them, and—

though the G-rated movies didn't get into the specifics of what happens in Disney bedrooms—surely perpetuated dated, centuries-old sexual scripts. Speaking your mind, speaking up for your needs, speaking out for your rights—heck, speaking at all—was not modeled either in Disney animation or mainstream live action Hollywood.

Fortunately for girls and young women today, television and movie roles have embraced more self-reliant, self-aware women. Even Disney female protagonists are different. The animated female stars of *Mulan*, *Frozen*, *Moana*, and *Encanto* consider options, contemplate actions, and take charge of their own destiny in incredible ways (learning to harness their powers, blatantly disregarding tradition to save their village, and restoring magical powers to their family members for starters), entirely unlike the princesses of Disney past. Even the 2023 live-action version of *The Little Mermaid* thankfully omitted Ursula's lines suggesting that men prefer women who don't speak.

Disney may have evolved its depiction of women from servile to progressive, but our greater society has not done nearly as good a job. Or rather, it has paid lip service to gender equality: We can vote, after all. We have more contraceptive options, we can apply to almost any college or university we want; women have held powerful government and corporate positions. But when push comes to shove, when members of our society are alone in a voting booth or in a bedroom with a partner, we resort to what we know; what we know, or what we have been conditioned to believe, is that women are in fact pleasers, givers, servers. Second fiddle to men. Why else would data support the continued wage gap, medical care gap, and other gaps that just don't make sense?[3] We know, deep inside, and then are reminded constantly, that power is for men. Both sexual power and sexual pleasure, too, are the domain of men. Sex might be *with* us, but it isn't *for* us, so we might as well just lay back and (pretend to) enjoy it. This is the essence of the Bedroom Gap.

One of the best quotes I've ever heard to describe the Bedroom Gap wasn't talking about it at all. It wasn't even focused on the United States. It comes from social scientist Deepa Narayan's TED talk, "7 Beliefs That Can Silence Women—and How to Unlearn Them." In the presentation, the international advisor on poverty, gender, and development talks about her experience interviewing six hundred educated, middle-class women, men, and children in India around one simple question: "What does it mean to be a *good* woman [or a good man] today?"[4]

In reflecting on the interviews, Narayan notes that nowadays, we think the world has changed, "but these external changes are extremely misleading. Because on the inside we have not changed." She goes on to say, "We don't need elastic women. We need elastic definitions." In other words, a "good woman" does not have to prioritize male needs, including male sexual pleasure. A "good woman" is not defined by her acting skills in making a man feel he is sexually pleasing her. A "good woman" does not have to believe that penis-in-vagina sex is the sole objective of intimacy.

Narayan's narrative can be used as a proxy for what women across the world experience in terms of midlife sex. Namely, they find that there are certain things expected of them and that it's a cause of great frustration when their bodies betray them, or when society privileges only patriarchal definitions of sex and pleasure to the detriment of all others.

While Narayan talks about Indian women, I've seen each of the seven beliefs she outlined in one form or another inside my practice. My patients—brilliant, accomplished women and self-proclaimed progressive thinkers—are distraught by their lack of sexual desire, their dry, less-enticing vaginas, and the belief that they *owe* their male partners good sex. They believe their own sexual pleasure is secondary to his. And as hard as they strive to make partner at their firm, to get tenure at their university, to become division head or department chair, they have already given up on the sexual victory for themselves. But this sexual settling, or pretending, is a pyrrhic victory.[5] For what women fail to realize is that by denying themselves sexual importance, by devaluing their own sexual pleasure, they diminish the experience for their partner. And this low level of sexual advocacy seems to be universal—for *women*.

My Princeton, New Jersey, clinic is down the street from a university that attracts scholars from all over the world, so my patients represent a wide array of sociocultural backgrounds; yet their problems with midlife sex are all the same, exposing and underscoring the universality of these issues. My professional experiences in the Middle East, South America, Africa, Australia, and Europe further confirm the universality of what I hear in my own clinic.

Are other countries more progressive about midlife women's health issues? For the most part, sadly, no. In a few countries—the United Kingdom, Australia, New Zealand, South Africa—testosterone for women is available by prescription, unlike in the United States where there is still no FDA-approved testosterone product on the market. (Interesting sidenote: Australia is also where, in the early 2000s, a female urologist was the first to truly study clitoral anatomy.) And yet, in the United States we are in the midst of what I call the Great Menopausal Awakening. As of 2025 more than twenty bills focused on menopause care and education have been introduced across thirteen states. California has passed the Menopause Care Equity Act, which requires insurance coverage for menopause treatments. Illinois Bill 0025 has created a Menopause Awareness Week in October. The legislation aims to make continuing medical education mandatory for physicians, make menopausal care affordable, and improve support in the workplace.[6]

Hey, it's hardly gender equality, but it's a start. What about progress on the sexual front in other countries? Certainly there are countries with more progressive views about sex. My friends and patients from several European countries, for example, encourage open dialogue about sex with their teenage and young adult children rather than just hoping teen sex doesn't happen. But as far as I can tell, grown-up sex talk, about things like dry vaginas, zero libido, and other midlife sexual issues for women remain shameful topics inside the United States and abroad.

Some of this is, without a doubt, cause for celebration. We are seeing progress—really, we are! But most of society still has a lot of work left to do with respect to acknowledging that humans continue to have sex for pleasure in middle age and beyond, and that sexual problems affecting this group are not addressed.

After thirty years of clinical practice and somewhere between eighty to one hundred thousand patient visits, I've heard different versions of the same story countless times. Women, mostly over forty, tell me they're broken. They tell me there's something wrong with them. And worst of all, many of them are convinced they're the only ones having these problems.

I've got news for you: You're not the only one. So many things are broken, from our education system to our medical system to how we approach biomedical research, from increasingly extreme and violent pornography to federal initiatives censoring words like *female* and *vagina* to the removal of funding of important NIH research on women's health. But *you* are not broken.

Feeling fired up right now? Good. Let's dig in. And then let's change the conversation and narrow the Bedroom Gap together. For ourselves, and for all the women who aren't here yet but who deserve better, because I promised Gloria.

PART ONE

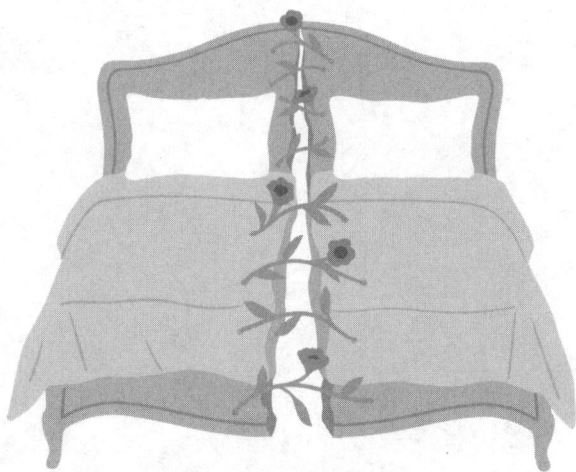

PART ONE

Chapter 1

What Happens to Our Lady Bits in Middle Age

I need Invisalign for my vagina!" exclaimed a boisterous fifty-something-year-old patient of mine. "It's more out of whack than my teenager's teeth!" "My vagina . . . has betrayed me," confessed another patient. "I think it's broken or something. No matter how much we try, sex just doesn't work. Nothing's getting in there. No matter what we do, I just can't get there these days."

I hear versions of this same story ten times a day in my practice: Middle-aged women who cannot have sex at all, who experience pain during sex, who lack desire, whose sex is devoid of pleasure, who have sex just to please their partner. Many of them are frustrated by an inability to have sex in the way they used to, and they feel so alone. They truly believe that theirs is a rare and shameful problem, unique to them. But this could not be further from the truth. What is going on here, and why do women feel so alone with their sexual issues?

Part of the reason is cultural shame, stigma, and silence—centuries old but persistent today—around all things related to female sex. In June 2012 Congresswoman Lisa Brown was commenting on a bill to limit abortion rights and said the word *vagina* (out loud, three times no less!); she was banned from the Michigan Statehouse. We don't even need to go back to previous centuries—this was just over a decade ago! Are we just super prudish?

There is a widespread squeamishness regarding females' mysterious nether regions. If women—and men for that matter—don't really understand their bodies and how they change—genitally, sexually, *functionally*—with age, then how are any of us supposed to know what is normal? If we can't publicly say the names for our anatomy in Congress, for God's sake, and don't understand the normal functioning of said anatomy, then how can we describe (to our partners, our friends, our clinicians) when we fear it is faltering?

Anatomy lessons are not the purpose of this book, though Chapter 2 will give you some pretty enlightening info on your lady bits and Chapter 7 contains a masturbation starter guide. But for now, let's just start by naming the problem. I believe the allergic reaction to and awkward repulsion elicited by female genitalia is a proxy for a fundamental lack of accurate knowledge, let alone acceptance, of what happens to women's bodies at all ages and stages, including after menopause.

(Hot) news flash: I've already noted that there are nearly eighty million menopausal women in the United States. Another two million American women a year, or *six thousand a day*, enter menopause. Worldwide, there are over a *billion* menopausal women, and another twenty-five million enter menopause each year.[1] Over a quarter of all females on the planet are over fifty, and 60 percent of them experience symptoms such as sexual pain, vaginal dryness, and loss of libido.[2] That is a *lot* of women, and most of them are suffering in silence. Crucially, the majority of these women—and their male partners—*don't connect the hormonal source of their hot flashes to the sexual symptoms they experience.* They don't realize that the dryness, tearing, pain, and loss of desire are by-products of hormonal deficiency.

GSM, the "New" Atrophy

Women bring lots of specific sexual issues to my office, but the culprit behind most of them is genitourinary syndrome of menopause (GSM), a mouthful of a term barely recognized by clinicians and unheard of in mainstream media. GSM is the current medical term for the constellation of symptoms that emerge when the genitals and bladder are deprived of estrogen. In the clinical discourse, GSM has replaced "vaginal atrophy," which experts felt didn't accurately describe the havoc wrought by the loss of estrogen on the rest of the region, including the labia, vulva, urethra, and bladder.

To be honest, I find both terms a bit pejorative. While "vaginal atrophy" makes me think of a mummified vagina, my issue with GSM is one of perception. I don't think women want to be labeled with a "syndrome" any more than a guy with erectile dysfunction (ED) wants to be labeled as having Floppy Penis Syndrome. On a positive note, and putting my lexical issues aside, the term GSM reflects the reality that *every* part of the female genitalia is affected by estrogen loss. Nothing is spared. Since GSM is the main reason behind the physical manifestations of the Bedroom Gap, it merits a quick explanation. It is important for us all to understand what happens to female bodies after menopause, why GSM is underdiagnosed and undertreated, and what we as advocates for better sexual relations can do about it.

Menopause:
What Really Happens

Many women, their partners, and even their doctors link menopause only to the end of menstrual periods; they don't fully understand that menopause "happens" when the ovaries stop producing steroid hormones, including progesterone, testosterone, and estrogen. This hormone drought in turn affects the many parts of the body that are estrogen dependent: the brain (estrogen receptors are found in numerous areas of the brain; brain fog anyone?); bones (this is why osteoporosis is largely a woman thing); muscle and joints (estrogen is an anti-inflammatory that prevents joint pain, arthritis, and muscle loss); fat (less estrogen means fat deposits in the abdomen more readily, not kidding); the heart (estrogen receptors are on the coronary arteries themselves, which may explain why heart disease in women increases dramatically after menopause); the bladder (now you know why your aunt always walked urgently to the mall bathroom); skin (turns out that wrinkles are not just from the sun); hair (yes, both hair loss on the scalp and new hairs on the face are related to menopause—thanks for nothing!); and of course the uterus and vagina. All these body parts and others suffer from hormonal abandonment.

The large number of estrogen-affected body systems is why menopause can have such frustratingly varied effects on women. The ovarian hormonal chaos of perimenopause, followed by hormonal absence in menopause, can present in different ways in different women, and in different ways at different times in the same woman! It is no wonder, then, that women often don't connect their wide-ranging issues—joint pains, palpitations, lethargy, and libido issues among others—to changes in their ovaries, a pair of tiny, almond-sized body parts they can't even feel.

Causes of GSM/Vaginal Atrophy

1. Natural menopause
2. Surgical menopause (which involves the removal of ovaries; removing the uterus does not equal surgical menopause!)
3. Menopause caused by chemo or radiation therapy
4. Postpartum/breastfeeding
5. Premature ovarian insufficiency (ovarian function stops before age forty, from genetic conditions, autoimmune disorders, infections, or possibly from exposure to toxins)
6. Medications, including:
   - drugs used in fertility care (GnRh or LHRH agonists)
   - oral contraceptives ("The Pill")
   - metformin

But even if women can't feel their ovaries, they *can* feel the havoc that estrogen loss wreaks on their genitourinary system. The genitourinary tract is loaded with estrogen receptors. Think of estrogen as pro-growth, pro-health, pro-female. It is sort of a growth hormone—essentially fertilizer for the body, mind, and maybe the soul—and when genital tissues are deprived of estrogen, a vaginal version of existential drought ensues. (Check out the fantastic animations a brilliant artist made for my TED talk to get a visual of what happens when the vagina is deprived of estrogen.)[3]

The vagina's strong, pliant premenopausal collagen is replaced in menopause by a weaker, lower quality version that breaks down more easily. Basically, our Neiman Marcus collagen gets swapped out for an IKEA-quality version. As a result, the ridges and clefts that allow the reproductive-age vagina to stretch with childbirth and accommodate penetrative sex flatten out. Worse, collagen isn't the only vaginal victim of aging; blood vessels also become scarce. In fact, blood vessel production grinds to a halt, and oh boy do we need them and miss them when they're gone. Blood vessels remove infection, carry nutrients, and leak fluid into the vagina when we get sexually aroused. As a result of this loss, vaginal color fades, moisture disappears, and sexually stimulated responses are blunted.

But wait, there's more. Estrogen loss affects the vaginal microbiome.[4] A balanced microbiome has been linked to both vaginal and bladder health. Changes in this unique biotic mix have been linked to the development of atrophy itself, as well as to bladder problems.

Finally, as if all these negative effects are not enough, in a God-must-be-a-man coup de grâce, the loss of estrogen leads to nerve endings for pleasure being unfairly replaced with those that sense pain. I kid you not.

The vulva and vagina "age" more quickly after menopause and not in the "with age comes wisdom" sort of way. Nobody comes to see me and announces she is thrilled with her new, middle-aged vagina. I told you the vagina "flattens" out—but what does that mean exactly? On a macro level, the vaginal opening narrows, the vaginal length shortens, and the elastic ridges, called rugae, smooth out, so the vagina loses its accordion-like ability to expand. Instead, it becomes inelastic, its walls paper thin and fragile. The dark pink color of vaginal youth fades to the pale pink of an unloved supermarket carnation and eventually to an anemic yellowish white. (I know, frightening but true.) The formerly plump outer labia begin to sag like two-day-old birthday balloons. The smooth, delicate inner lips, the labia minora, thin and shrivel, and the clitoris shrinks so much that in some women it becomes barely visible.

When I examine women with severe GSM, I can barely insert the tip of my pinky finger into their vagina, never mind a speculum. Attempting to insert anything inside them results in reflexive wincing and tightening of pelvic floor muscles. This very understandable reaction also has a somewhat off-putting name: vaginismus. Clinically, it is the involuntary tensing of muscles around the vagina. It is common—between 5 and 17 percent of all women experience this—and can occur even if a woman has previously tolerated vaginal penetration.

In women with even more pronounced GSM, the labia minora actually fuse together to further close the caliber of the vaginal opening. Ouch! When fusion occurs at the top-most portion of the labia, it covers over the clitoris and further diminishes clitoral sensation and sexual pleasure. This is called clitoral phimosis, and it can be a sexual disaster. In severe cases of GSM, the labia are riddled with cuts, tears, fissures; even gentle pressure splits apart paper-thin vulvar tissue, which sometimes bleeds to light touch.

What I can't see when I examine patients is a cruel reduction in pleasure-sensing nerve endings paired with more receptors that perceive pain. Even our own bodies are giving in to the notion that sex after menopause is more pain than pleasure. What fresh hell is this, indeed! No wonder the women who come to see me can't get excited about sex anymore. Everything that used to turn them on doesn't seem to work anymore. Is it their partners, or is their body betraying them?

What Happens During Arousal?

We can better understand some of the bedroom concerns menopausal women face if we take a look at what happens—or doesn't—during sexual arousal. It turns out that arousal has pretty profound effects on the female genitals. When we get turned on, neurochemicals in the brain communicate marching orders to the genitalia. Arousal causes shifts in blood flow, resulting in swelling and a deepening in color of the labia and the lower third of the vagina; it also encourages lubrication, which makes penetration more comfortable. During arousal, the vagina itself lengthens and dilates in anticipation of penetration. Muscles around the clitoris relax to allow blood to rush into the clitoral tip. The clitoris—the female homologue to the penile shaft—becomes swollen and actually elevates toward the pubic bone. Our own version of an erection!

Let's break this down a little further.

How We Get Wet and Why We Don't, or You Can't Fake Moisture

Of all the unwelcome vaginal changes that women experience with estrogen loss, dryness tends to be the most maddening. Perhaps this is because if a woman cannot lubricate with arousal, she fears it is a signal to her partner that she is not attracted to him/her, or not interested, or just not in the mood. You can't fake moisture. Like an erection, it is there or it isn't, and when it's absent, both parties know it. And vaginal dryness often makes for painful sex, which can kill your sex life all by itself.

Lubrication, the more formal term for "getting wet" from sexual arousal, happens when fluid within blood vessels seeps from behind the vaginal walls into the vagina. Our on-demand vaginal moisture is made of ultra-filtrated blood, which is actually mostly water mixed with a few proteins and some vaginal cells. Estrogen also helps with lubrication by facilitating the enzymatic reactions that allow the process to happen, as well as by promoting blood vessel growth. Side note: Vibration from vibrators does this too! So can erotic stimuli, such as looking at sexual images or reading erotica.

During sex, stress on the vaginal tissue stimulates nerves, which produce chemical signals to open the blood vessels, and the resulting fluid seeps across the vaginal walls. The more blood vessels there are, the more opportunities for flow of moisture into the vagina.

The good news is that the vagina does not rely solely on its vasculature for wetness: It has two pairs of lube systems for added slippery wetness.

The Beautiful and Sexy Glands

The other system working to get us wet—contributing yet more icing on the cake of vaginal lubrication during arousal—involves two sets of glands, the Bartholin's and Skene's, or as I call them, the Beautiful and Sexy (B and S) glands, which are perfectly located near the opening of the vagina. The glands are important for good sex because they secrete mucus and fluid to make the vagina slicker, penetration more facile, and sex more fun. Think of the shape of the vaginal opening as a clock. The paired Bartholin's glands are located at five and seven o'clock, right at the sweet spot where a penis first enters the vagina, while the pair of Skene's glands are located at eleven and one o'clock, flanking the opening to the bladder. With sexual arousal, the Bartholin's glands secrete mucus to lubricate the vagina; the Skene's glands secrete fluid around the urethral opening, making the whole genital milieu more moist and slippery.

Importantly, due to their location near the opening of the vagina, the two pairs of glands ensure that the vagina is lubricated and penetration is helped right from the beginning. These glands are key to comfortable sex, and when menopause deprives them of estrogen, they just don't work as well, making less moisture and less mucus.

Welcome to Church: The Vestibule

The third factor important for comfortable sex is the health of the vaginal opening, known as the vestibule. Pain located at the vestibule is the most common complaint related to a specific area. When a woman tells me that sex hurts, the number one culprit is this type of pain. An elastic, well-estrogenized, well-lubricated, healthy vestibule is tantamount to comfortable sex.

So Many Things Can Go Wrong

As you can see, there is a lot going on "down there" when one is sexually aroused, and that means a lot can go wrong. When a lack of estrogen causes a lack of lubrication or elasticity and subsequent pain, the whole symphony of sexual arousal can fall apart. The impact of a given sexual response or lack thereof can be huge. A limp penis sends a message: "You are not attracted to me. You aren't turned on. Something is wrong." A dry vagina sends the same message. It is not exaggeration to say that estrogen deficiency is responsible for many an affair, breakups, separation, divorce, and can be blamed for much of the relationship discord behind the Bedroom Gap.

Even the Bladder Needs Estrogen

If few women link their vaginal and sexual issues to a lack of estrogen, even fewer can comprehend that the deficiency causes urinary issues. Like many other parts of the body, estrogen receptors are found aplenty in the bladder, but it is estrogen's effect *in the vagina* that keeps us from getting UTIs. It turns out that estrogen is responsible not only for the health of the vaginal tissue itself but also for the functional health and balance of the vaginal microbiome, which in turn keeps the bladder healthy. (Interesting sidenote: Imbalances in the vaginal microbiome have been linked to everything from premature birth to HPV and the development of cervical cancer.)

Estrogen and the Vaginal Microbiome

Unlike in today's university student bodies and boardroom composi-
tions, we don't want diversity in our vaginal microbiome. We want relatively few species, predominantly Lactobacillus. High levels of estrogen
make a lactobacillus-loaded microbiome. When estrogen levels drop,
there are fewer Lactobacilli to produce lactic acid. This shifts the vaginal
pH and upsets the makeup of the whole bacterial neighborhood.

How do estrogen and a healthy microbiome prevent UTIs? Our
bladder sits nestled against the lower part of our uterus. It empties via
a single drainage tube at its bottom, called the urethra. The urethra
opens out into the world right at the worst possible spot, just where a
penis thrusts with penetration. The urethral opening is along the top
wall of the vagina just below the clitoris, and it is pretty hard to avoid
contact with the urethral opening when you are inserting a tampon
or a vibrator or a penis or pretty much anything into the vagina. This
means the vagina needs to be healthy around the urethral opening,
and it is estrogen that keeps plenty of good bacteria like Lactobacilli around the area to keep the infection-causing bad bacteria from
getting into the urethra where they then have access to the bladder.
When estrogen levels go down, the vaginal microbiome changes and
there are fewer protective Lactobacilli to guard the opening to the
bladder.

Other Ways We Can Help with GSM Symptoms

Lasers and Probiotics

There are other ways to reduce UTIs. Vaginal and oral probiotics are
getting a lot of attention, as some studies suggest they are effective
at promoting a good microbiome and reducing urinary infections.
Vaginal treatments with CO_2 lasers may reduce UTI occurrence by

creating small painless microdots that act as "injuries" to the vaginal tissue; this triggers blood vessel and collagen production. The increase in blood vessels along the top wall of the vagina, which is just under the bladder and urethra, improves blood flow and helps with bladder (and sexual) health. Such lasers were brought to the United States in 2015 (by me!) and are a nonmedication alternative to vaginal estrogen; in experienced hands, they are safe and effective. But treatments are not insurance covered and can be costly, so widespread use is unlikely. Moreover neither probiotics nor laser therapy has been shown to be superior to the proven urinary health benefits of vaginal or systemic estrogen, which leads to a nice bump in the levels of Lactobacilli and other good guy bacterial species. Our vaginal microbiome becomes balanced and protective once again. Urinary infections magically decrease. Ta-da!

Ospemifene

Besides vaginal estrogen and CO_2 laser treatments, prescription medications can reverse GSM. Ospemifene, a nonhormonal oral medication, has been FDA-approved for treatment of GSM symptoms. This selective estrogen receptor modifier (SERM) selectively turns on estrogen receptors in some tissues (in this case, vagina, bladder, and bone) while turning off or having no effect on estrogen receptors in other body parts. Because of its positive effect on bone, it may be a nice option for women with GSM who also have family history of osteoporosis or have osteoporosis or osteopenia themselves. It seems ospemifene also has a positive effect on the vaginal microbiome, providing further relief from GSM.

Progesterone

Does progesterone play a role in GSM? The simple answer is "no." Progesterone receptors are notably absent in the external and internal female genitalia and play no role in the development or treatment of GSM. But that shouldn't take away from the incredibly vital role progesterone plays for women of all ages.

Although it doesn't benefit the vagina itself per se, progesterone does have many functions throughout a woman's reproductive lifespan. It is important in regulating menstruation and supports early pregnancy. During our reproductive years, progesterone prepares the endometrium—the tissue lining the womb—for the embryo to implant. (Think of preparing a bed with a nice thick downy duvet.)

Progesterone also stimulates glands in the endometrium to secrete nutrients for the embryo. A duvet plus a healthy breakfast in bed! This amazing hormone also keeps the uterine muscle from contracting, thus preventing miscarriage. The etymology of the word ("pro": favoring and "gest": gestation, or pregnancy) tells it all. If there is no conception in a given menstrual cycle, the progesterone-filled cyst in the ovary, the corpus luteum, breaks down and progesterone levels fall. The endometrium thins and sheds, which we call a period. I guess you could say that each month we create a hormonally grown duvet for an embryo. If there is no pregnancy that month, we literally throw out our endometrial duvet.

Progesterone could also be called "pro*sleep*erone," since it promotes sleep by producing GABA, short for gamma aminobutyric acid. GABA is a neurotransmitter in the brain that dampens the activity of neurons, making them less excitable, less responsive to stimulation. This produces a calming effect that reduces anxiety and promotes restful sleep. Less progesterone in menopause means less GABA. Perhaps this is why many women in perimenopause and menopause don't sleep well.

Progesterone also acts in opposition to estrogen to limit the growth of the uterine lining, called the endometrium, and to prevent hyperplasia and cancer from developing in the uterus; this is why women with a uterus need progesterone as well as estrogen when they use hormones after menopause. Otherwise we would be "feeding" the uterus estrogen, and the growth of the lining cells would go unchecked. This is also why being overweight is a risk factor for uterine cancer. Fat cells are a repository for estrogen; extra body fat means exposing your uterus to extra estrogen, but in menopause there is no progesterone to offset it. Without the progesterone to offset the estrogen-fueled growth, the endometrium can grow excessively and abnormally. Think Girls Gone Wild minus the tequila shots.

Testosterone

Testosterone, on the other hand, *is* a major player in the vulvovaginal world, and its loss from menopause impacts our vulvar, vaginal, and sexual health—really, it impacts our whole body. It is hard to overstate testosterone's beneficial effects for women, even though it is thought of as a "male" hormone.

You might be wondering, "What is testosterone, the quintessential male hormone, doing in the vagina?" The answer is embryological. Every human fetus starts out female by default. (Yes, really!) Fetal genitalia are undifferentiated until around six to seven weeks of (uterine) age when, if the fetus has a Y chromosome, the testicles develop. Around nine weeks of fetal age, testosterone is produced, which moves the masculinization ball forward. In essence, the testes are just external versions of ovaries, except they need a cooler environment and so were moved outside the body in the process of evolution, protected by the thick, tough skin of the scrotum.

Testosterone works hard to keep life down there fun and functional for females. When our ovaries stop producing testosterone, the labia become dry, thin, delicate; the puffy fat pads of the labia majora that function as cushions disappear, opening the possibility for discomfort with sports or sex. The luxuriant premenopausal vulva becomes hollow, sagging, deflated. (Sorry, depressing, but true . . .)

Testosterone receptors abound on the clitoris, in the lower third of the vagina, and at the vaginal opening, so when GSM develops and testosterone levels fall, orgasms become less intense and many women have pain at the vestibule. Testosterone is also responsible for the protective pubic hair women try so hard to groom or remove.[5] When testosterone levels fall during and after menopause, the thickness, color, and density of pubic hair changes. Hairs become softer and shorter. If you don't want the sparse patchy look of menopausal pubic hair, topical testosterone or DHEA creams can partially reactivate hair growth, and some women regain hair density and thickness in three to six months of use.

Testosterone keeps the external genitals strong and healthy and the whole genital system sexually responsive. The hormone helps to maintain the shape and resiliency of the larger outer "lips," the labia majora, so we can go horseback riding and hit the Peloton and have sex. It keeps the delicate thin labia minora excitable, so they can swell and change color with sexual arousal. It keeps the clitoris responsive to touch and pressure. It facilitates elasticity of the vaginal opening, which can then stretch to allow tampons and toys to be inserted comfortably.

So, if the tissues harmed by the deteriorating effects of GSM respond to testosterone, why not just use a testosterone vaginal tablet, ring, suppository, or cream? Or why don't we blend testosterone with the topical estrogen creams used to help with GSM in these specific areas? Quite simply, there is no FDA-approved, commercially available topical testosterone formulation for women in the United States. This is not true in other countries, but in the United States, there is still no available testosterone formulation for women. This has always seemed ludicrous to me, as well as to most of my colleagues who specialize in menopause and sexual medicine. (Later in the book, we will uncover the pharmaceutical, financial, and sociocultural reasons for this.)

Hormone: The Dirty Word

Unfortunately, there are widespread concerns among women and many clinicians about the safety of hormonal therapies. *Hormone* has become a feared and dirty word in medical therapy. Many women have heard that hormone therapy is used to treat GSM, but they have a lot of concerns. Often patients come to me to discuss the idea, but they tend to open the conversation with "I'm not really comfortable using anything hormonal. I don't want to get cancer."

Think about this. Would a clinician risk their medical license and reputation to treat a patient with something known to cause cancer? I am pretty sure the answer is a resounding *no*. Let's clear something up: The (now debunked) link between cancer risk and hormone therapy came from a study launched in 1991, with results released in 2002, which examined among other things the cancer risk of oral, systemic therapy. That study, the Women's Health Initiative (WHI), did not examine the risks of vaginal estrogen, which is perhaps the best option to treat GSM. The hormonal preparations currently available by prescription in the United States to treat GSM are *vaginal, not oral*. They are well-studied, FDA-approved, and have not been shown to cause cancer. The hormonal prescription options we offer to help women with GSM symptoms have been well vetted and are extremely safe and quite effective.[6]

Ignorance Isn't Bliss

As we age, the kinds of vaginal, vulvar, and bladder changes we've been discussing in this book come as a surprise to many women and their partners. Why? Because just like our reluctance to discuss female pleasure, we as a society don't talk about "women stuff."

To make matters worse, physicians and other women's health care clinicians are not well trained in either menopause or female sexual issues, and many clinicians are embarrassed to discuss sex at all with patients. Sadly, most of them aren't even familiar with the term *GSM* and very few understand how it develops, think to ask about it, or know how to treat it.

GSM should be something all women and their partners, not to mention their clinicians, know about; yet it remains a taboo subject, a dirty secret, a mystery. So many women over the years have come into my office believing their vaginal atrophy was a rare freak of nature, a phenomenon that has happened only to them, and of which they should be ashamed. They never learned about GSM from their mothers or friends, from health class, or from watching TV and movies. No film director suggests an actress swap the sweaty thralls of orgasmic pleasure for the wincing pain of GSM sex. Given the lack of screen time and lack of discourse within society on the subject, one would be forgiven for thinking GSM a rare disease.

But GSM is common. Over half of the nearly eighty million menopausal women in the United States and half of the one billion menopausal women globally have GSM. That means that at least five hundred million women *right now* are enduring genital or urinary symptoms that are largely treatable.

Many shows use menopause for laughs and avoid giving this major midlife shift in mental, physical, and sexual health more than a wink and a nod. I don't expect Hollywood to become a mouthpiece for clinical medicine, but a little peek into what the sexual effects of menopause can be like could go a long way in terms of letting women know what is normal and that it is okay to talk about what you're experiencing with your gal pals, your partner, and your health care provider.

So Many of Us

As the enormous baby boomer generation faces menopause and women are living longer, the sheer number of women with postmenopausal sexual issues has increased. As already noted, an estimated six thousand women in the United States become menopausal every single day, and at least half of those women have or will have symptoms of GSM. Hear that? That is the sound of a lot of Bedroom Gaps widening all over the country, and the problem is not being addressed. Nearly the entirety of the two tranches of boomers, ages 58–67 and 68–76 years old, are already menopausal; even half of the Gen Xers, now aged 46–57, are menopausal, given that the average age of menopause is 51.5.

In case you need more convincing, let me underscore the prevalence of GSM symptoms. In one study of nine hundred women, 84 percent reported vaginal dryness, painful intercourse, reduced capacity for orgasm, and increased bladder and vaginal infections only six years after their periods stopped. To make matters worse, the problems resulting from GSM are *chronic and progressive*. This progressive deterioration may lead women to think their genital atrophy is not related to menopause, since most other menopause symptoms eventually resolve. By the time women are in their late fifties, the hormonal chaos has tempered. Menopause-related mood changes, temperature intolerance, and weight increase have usually steadied. But the sexual problems can persist long after these other, more recognizable symptoms have lessened.

One of my patients, Anna, had long since stopped having hot flashes; she thought she had "finished with menopause" and that her bladder and sexual issues were due to "something else." For Anna, sex was so painful it had become impossible. She worried that there was something uniquely wrong with her—maybe something was damaged or even abnormal in her body. "I think it's just me," she suggested. "Something's broken down there," she said and nervously giggled when she came to me with her concerns.

Sex remains an awkward topic to bring up for most women. In a National Poll on Healthy Aging, only 17 percent of men and women discuss sexual issues with a clinician.[7] The same percentage of respondents said that if they had a sexual issue, they would not feel comfortable discussing it with anyone. That is, *almost one in five women won't discuss their sexual problems with anyone.*

GSM is a huge quality of life issue. When Anna was in my office, she confessed that her recurrent urinary tract infections—one of which occurred after she tried to have penetrative sex—have made her afraid to have sex at all. Additionally, the tightness and dryness and the throbbing pain she feels for a few days after attempts at sex have left her feeling frustrated. "I feel like a disabled person. Like I am a hundred years old," she told me. "I feel like this shouldn't bother me; it shouldn't be a big deal. But it is. For me and for my husband."

Of course it is a big deal! And this was something I could help her with. I recommended she start with a prescription for vaginal estrogen. When I saw her again three months later, Anna's "broken vagina" was almost magically improved. She was able to have enjoyable, penetrative sex; she was able to feel the production of her own moisture; she was able again to orgasm; and the UTIs had not recurred. Three months of vaginal estrogen had restored not only health to her vagina but health to her self-esteem and to her relationship.

GSM affects the quality of a woman's life in so many ways. The *Real Women's Views of Treatment Options for Menopausal Vaginal Changes* (REVIVE) study is a survey of 3,046 women in the United States. The findings showed that GSM symptoms had negative effects on multiple parameters of a woman's life. They led to loss of intimacy for 85 percent of respondents, detracted from enjoyment of sex for 59 percent, interfered with their relationship for 47 percent, negatively

affected sleep for 29 percent, and adversely affected the general enjoyment of life for 27 percent.

The Bedroom Gap Is Global

These issues are not only an American problem. Listening to women
from diverse backgrounds and different countries over the past thirty
years has confirmed for me the universality of the female sexual experience, replete with frustration and acceptance. It also says a lot about
what women think is expected of them, and what men presume
about sex. Luz-Maria, in Mendoza, Argentina, has regular sex with
her husband even though it is "extremely painful," because she feels
obliged. "What kind of Latin man doesn't want to have sex? I can't
expect him to give that up."

Celeste, from Brisbane, Australia, loves her husband, Simon,
she just has no interest in sex. She figures having sex is an insurance
policy to "keep him around, to keep him from straying. You know,
men have needs. If he's not getting those needs met at home, he might
look elsewhere." Maryam, a woman in Abu Dhabi, told me she keeps
a stick by her bed. During coitus, she grabs it and squeezes the sharp
areas of the stick to distract herself from the pain of penetration. She
had borne seven children and her husband had two other, younger,
wives, as was customary in her community. "I hoped that he would
take interest only in the beds of the younger wives," she said, "so I
wouldn't have to deal with the pain, but he always came back to my
bed. I was honored, and proud that he still wanted me, but I knew
that also meant more pain, and sometimes cuts and tears and bleeding as well."

Some years ago I was asked to speak about sexual health at a
Women's Health conference in Dubai. The hotel ballroom was full,
with five hundred clinicians from all over the Middle East in atten-
dance. Rows of men in full length white *dishdashas* occupied most of

the room while the women lined the back wall dressed in long, flowing black *abayas*. All of the women wore the *hijab* headdress in variations: Some sported only the *shayla*, a light scarf covering the hair; others wore a *gishwa*, a light semitransparent veil that covered the face. A few wore a *niqab*, an opaque cloth covering the face entirely with an opening for the eyes. When my talk ended, about three hundred hands went up. It seemed everyone had questions. Had I done such a lousy job that nobody understood my talk? The gyn-oncologist slated to give the next lecture stood up and took the microphone that had been set up for questions.

"I have been attending this conference since it began, and we have never had a lecture that dared to really talk about sexual health," the speaker said. "The clinicians at this conference need to hear what you have to say. We get no formal training in matters of sex. I yield my time to you, Dr. Sophocles, so you can answer all these questions and tell us all more about how to talk with our patients about this awkward but important topic." I was stunned, grateful, embarrassed, and proud all at once. The audience members rushed up for their turn at the microphone like I was giving away Taylor Swift tickets. Even an hour later, the questions kept coming and the discussion remained lively.

Because of the cultural barriers in their societies, these clinicians had been taught even less than their American counterparts, and their patients were even less comfortable talking about these subjects. Sexual problems exist everywhere—GSM doesn't care where you live. The *Vaginal Health: Insights, Views and Attitudes* (VIVA) online survey queried 3,520 postmenopausal women in six countries. Seventy-five percent felt their vaginal symptoms negatively affected their lives. Among the US respondents, 80 percent reported their vaginal discomfort had a negative effect on their lives; 75 percent said it negatively affected sexual intimacy; 68 percent reported feeling less sexual; 36 percent said it made them feel old; 33 percent said it had negative effects on their marriage/relationship; 26 percent said it negatively affected their self-esteem; and 25 percent reported an overall lower quality of life.[8]

GSM is a universal, common, and miserable experience, and it affects so many more people than you might think. For example, GSM is not unique to menopausal women. Sadly, it can occur in any woman with estrogen deficiency, irrespective of age and cause. Loss of estrogen may also result from surgical menopause, in which the ovaries are removed, with or without a hysterectomy.

Postpartum and breastfeeding women experience an estrogen drop much like menopause, and as a result, GSM can develop in these young, otherwise healthy women. It can also develop in athletes, dancers, women with eating disorders, and other women with a very low body fat content. Then there are women who experience an immunologic-caused premature menopause, called primary ovarian insufficiency (POI), in which the lack of systemic estrogen affects bones, heart, skin, and of course the vagina. But let's be honest—we are all being inadequately treated by our medical industry. It appears that the biopharma industry has found it neither useful nor profitable enough to merit the research and development of treatments for a life condition that 100 percent of women and 50 percent of the planet's population experiences.

The other half of the global population doesn't have to worry that their issues with sexual aging are being ignored; their problems remain front and center in both doctor's offices and the pharmaceutical industry. Thirty years ago, Big Pharma rocked the world of sexual health—on behalf of *men*. I mean, who hasn't heard of Viagra? A huge boon for men and their penises—but how much did women benefit from this medical breakthrough? Not. At. All. How come Big Pharma hasn't figured out how to help women in the same way?

Chapter 2

✿

Sex, Sexism, and the Little Blue Pill

Jane and her partner, Sam, came to see me on a blustery Thursday. Jane had heard me on Sirius XM talking about female sexual issues, and they drove sixteen hours to talk with me. (Unfortunately for Jane and Sam, this was before the COVID pandemic accelerated telemedicine!) They both wore jeans, flannel shirts, and boots. Jane's long, straight hair was dark brown, thoroughly streaked with gray, and her blue eyes looked tired, sad. If she was hopeful, she kept that emotion well hidden. Sam had a beautiful mustache and a weather-beaten look to him.

They thanked me for seeing them and came right to the point. "We can't have sex. We haven't been able to for eight years. And we want to. She wants to," Sam stated. Jane nodded, pursed her lips, opened her mouth, then closed it again. What did she want to add? "I think I'm broken down there or something," she offered. What Jane shared later in the visit, after her exam while Sam waited in the waiting room, was that Sam's recent Viagra use—he was finding erections a bit challenging even with masturbation—had made an already problematic situation even worse. His ability to have on-demand, prolonged erections increased his desire to have penetrative sex, but due to the pain she was experiencing, their sexual interactions left her feeling inept, inadequate, and "broken."

Jane's sexual pain, which seemed to be caused by GSM, had thus far gone untreated. Sam's inability to maintain an erection, on the other hand, had been well taken care of. Why is that?

As we age, many body functions deteriorate: vision, hearing, reflexes. In most men, erectile function diminishes as well.[1] As we learned in Chapter 1, for at least half of women, aging brings the genital deterioration of collagen, depletion of blood vessels, and reduction of pleasure-sensing nerve endings, which impair sexual function in many ways. For couples of roughly the same age, sexual changes often occurred in tandem. You had sex together. You got older together. You had less sex, or different sex, or sexual difficulties *together*. Maybe because such changes occur for both sexes and at roughly the same pace, there has always been a tacit acceptance of this facet of aging.

But when the availability of medications for sexual dysfunction such as Viagra returned male erectile vigor to its youth, it left women without any similar ability to turn back the clock on genital health. Women were suddenly left to sexually age out, alone.

We as a society just don't value enhancing female sexual response, which is reflected in the lack of funding, research, development, and approval of viable effective medical options for women.

We have already discussed how sex has historically been and remains androcentric in its aim—primarily as an act for female-burdened reproduction and for male pleasure. And guess what? Viagra and other medications like it have simply increased the androcentricity of sex. While there has always been a Bedroom Gap, this midlife discrepancy between sexual desire in men and women, with all the itinerant sociological, physiological, and cultural influences, medical therapy for erectile dysfunction or enhancement tipped the scales of the bedroom imbalance. In short, Viagra has widened the Bedroom Gap even further.

When Viagra launched in 1998, the earliest male boomers were turning fifty. It should come as no surprise that they were very eager to embrace the opportunity to rejuvenate their middle-aged sex lives, to conquer their ED, and to recapture the erections of their youth. The Little Blue Pill, nicknamed "The Pfizer Riser," sold a billion dollars' worth of sexual excitement in its first year, not only reinvigorating intimacy all over the United States but revitalizing the pharmaceutical industry. Viagra's was the most successful prescription drug launch in history.[2] By 2002 Pfizer was the fifth most profitable corporation in the United States.[3] Viagra became the fastest-selling drug ever produced. In the United States alone, Viagra has been prescribed more than thirty-nine million times to over twenty million patients by over three hundred thousand physicians. It continues, despite numerous competitors, to generate nearly three million prescriptions yearly. Globally, seven Viagra tablets are dispensed every second, or 25,200 tablets every hour.

Did this drug discovery/marketing coup represent the pathologization of a variant of normal? Or a safe improvement in quality of life? Or the commercialization of prescription medicine? Probably it was a blend of all three—product, promise, and profit.

The Little Blue Pill didn't even begin as an erection cure. It was developed as a cardiology medication that had the surprising side effect of prolonging erections. Pfizer quickly scrapped the idea of promoting Viagra for lowering blood pressure when the company realized it had stumbled upon something that would change even more lives and please both patients and shareholders.

The development of a pill to treat ED was indeed novel, but the evolution from successful drug launch to cultural phenomenon was a product of the perfect alignment of several factors. According to Meika Loe, author of *The Rise of Viagra: How the Little Blue Pill Changed Sex in America*, "Viagra's emergence in the late twentieth century can be distilled down to five shifting sets of social circumstances: 1. medical expansion, 2. scientific and technological innovation, 3. pharmaceutical deregulation and expansion, 4. cultural and demographic shifts in gender and aging, and 5. increasing scientific and popular attention to sexuality and sexual dissatisfaction."[4]

A more public interest in sex may have spurred research that led to the development of the first birth control pill, Enovid, in 1960. Suddenly women had agency over their reproductive health. They could control pregnancy, and sex could be for fun, not merely for reproduction. The advent of "the pill" was a harbinger of what was to come: the cultural merging of medicine and technology with sociocultural desires. From this point on, the purpose of medical treatments was not merely to cure disease or to prolong life but to refine and enhance the quality of health, including reproductive and sexual health. Researchers William Masters and Virginia Johnson became famous in the 1960s for their groundbreaking work on the physiology of human sexuality. The 1960s and '70s saw a sexual revolution that primed the pump, so to speak, for the approval of Viagra in the 1990s.

Viagra's Perfect Storm of Success

So, which came first, the diagnosis or the med? Well, surprise surprise, there's more to the story.

Medical Expansion

Medical expansion refers to the medicalization of previously nonmedical life situations, such as baldness, depression, ADHD, PMS, menopause, and erectile dysfunction. Does the availability of medical therapies for these conditions lead to more frequent diagnosis? It seems so. For example, as ADHD diagnoses rose in the 1990s, more meds became available. As awareness grew, more parents and patients asked clinicians about symptoms, which led to more testing and more diagnoses being made and, in turn, more prescriptions written.

Which begs the question: Are there really more people with ADHD now or just more people aware of meds for ADHD, seeking a diagnosis and prescription to "fix" a student who can't stay focused in class?[5] Regardless of the causes, we know awareness of the condition has skyrocketed in recent years. During the COVID lockdown, for example, there were 11.4 billion TikTok views on #ADHD—by 2024, just four years later, these had increased to thirty-six billion.[6] In the UK, ADHD medication prescriptions increased by 800 percent between 2000 and 2015, and the trend toward increased prescriptions, especially in adult women, has continued.[7] This may be due to increased awareness of the diagnosis by the public and clinicians, increased medication options on offer, or both.

Do clinicians succumb to overdiagnosing because a drug rep has bought them lunch and left samples? Do physicians feel pressure to prescribe if a patient requests a medication she heard about on a podcast or a TV ad and wants to leave a visit with that prescription?

Viagra's explosion into American consciousness was an early example of the medicalization of a diagnosis, in this case erectile dysfunction. As more and more people heard about Viagra and went in to see their doctors, ED diagnoses and prescriptions went up. At the time of its approval in 1998, Viagra had the fastest initial sales growth of any prescription product following its launch, and as advertising

reached consumers and awareness reached clinicians, sales continued to increase, peaking in 2012 at over $2 billion in annual sales.
Even in 2019, after the approval of generic Viagra known as sildenafil,
Viagra still generated around $500 million in US revenue.[8] Medical
expansion of this condition, along with many others, was occurring
in the United States at the same time that our enormous middle-aged
populace was looking to optimize health and well-being.

Demographics

Historically, the timing of Viagra's launch was demographically perfect. Baby boomers born after the end of the Second World War were
rapidly reaching middle age in the late nineties. In the United States,
approximately seventy-nine million babies were born during the
baby boom, of which roughly forty million were males. The dramatic
increase in births helped lead to exponential rises in the demand for
consumer products, suburban homes, automobiles, roads, and ser-
vices, a phenomenon that persisted into the 1990s. The middle-aged
boomers were a perfect target audience for Viagra. They had lived in
relatively peaceful times and had disposable income; they wanted
to live longer and to stay physically—and sexually—fit. They had a
young and virile president, Bill Clinton, and many had been young
and virile teens during the presidency of another young and virile
president, JFK. Both presidents had well-known robust sexual appetites, at a time when male sexual conquests were equated with power,
youth, even health. (This, of course, was way before #MeToo and
before anyone thought to ask about the sexual needs of the women
brought into the White House for JFK's dalliances, or about whether
Monica Lewinsky's sexual needs were being met during her affair
with Bill Clinton.)

Sex was for male pleasure, and men were entitled to sex in
whatever context they were able to get it. The large demographic

numbers of the male boomers meant purchasing power, which did not go unnoticed by the for-profit visionaries in the pharmaceutical industry.

Big Pharma Becomes Powerful

In the late 1990s pharmaceutical companies were becoming increasingly powerful—at the time, there were more pharma lobbyists than congressmen in Washington, DC—and Big Pharma was among the most profitable sectors in industry. These companies' increasing power in Washington also extended to the FDA, where pressure could be applied to accelerate the approval of medication.

The growth and profitability of Big Pharma also enabled the funding of research. As of 2003, nearly 75 percent of funding for clinical trials came from industry rather than government.[9] An article published in 2020 studied the decreasing percentage of government research funding and found that between 2000 and 2017, the percentage of basic research funded by the federal government declined from 58 to 42 percent.[10] In short, in the early twenty-first century, the development of new drugs shifted from academic universities to pharmaceutical companies. This shift changed incentives in drug development from curing disease to pleasing shareholders through strong product sales. Nowhere was the commercialization of medicine more blatant than in the launch of Viagra.

Medical Diagnoses: From Psychogenic to Physiologic Causes

Executives at Pfizer had a quandary. They had stumbled upon a drug that could treat erectile dysfunction—a potential gold mine, they knew. But how to launch a drug for impotence, a condition that was embarrassing, private, even shameful? It was a topic even physicians were loath to bring up, much less patients. Pfizer needed a spokesperson who Americans could trust on this taboo subject. And so, when Pfizer tapped respected senator and war veteran Bob Dole to speak about his issues with ED following surgery for prostate cancer, he was calm and strong. His mainstream television appearance felt less like a commercial—Viagra was never even mentioned—and more like the farewell address of a military general. Dole urged male viewers to find the *courage* to learn about ED.

Initially the drug wasn't marketed for everyone, just those men *brave* enough to confront impotence, a term laced with shame and failure. Dole's words were carefully chosen and his performance was calm, powerful, brave. He was speaking to the *strong* American males who had the *courage* to discuss this delicate problem with their doctors. It was a call to action.

The Bob Dole ad became iconic and not only destigmatized ED but opened the door to direct-to-consumer (DTC) advertising for prescription medication. DTC advertising had long been prohibited, but the ban was lifted in August 1997, just six months before Viagra was launched. After the campaign kicked off, the public started going (in droves!) to their clinicians with a request for a prescription medication they learned about on TV.

Pfizer's masterful marketing team and media-savvy clinical consultants succeeded in converting "impotence"—which had previously been thought of as an unfortunate by-product of aging or, even worse, a psychology-based sexual inadequacy—to a simple, less embarrassing, plumbing problem: "erectile dysfunction." ED was a mechanical problem that could be easily cured with a pill.[11]

The shift from the term impotence to ED reflects the prevailing medical trend of the times, whereby causes for medical diagnoses shifted from psychogenic to physiological. The neurochemical explanation for depression and the emergence of SSRIs such as Prozac is a perfect example. Doctors could more comfortably prescribe and consumers more readily accept taking a pill for a serotonin deficit than for depression, a "mental health condition" with associated shame and stigma.

Pfizer ads for Viagra did the same: They didn't show depressed, weak, or psychologically unwell men lamenting their inability to get or maintain an erection. Instead, they highlighted healthy, mostly white, heterosexual men over forty who have otherwise wonderful lives but have a minor, treatable medical issue.

Dr. Irwin Goldstein, Pfizer's articulate and media-savvy clinical consultant, is credited with converting the term impotence to erectile dysfunction. A respected researcher, Goldstein carried out studies on ED and Viagra for Pfizer, including a 1994 study that brought public attention to the prevalence of male sexual dysfunction. Between Bob Dole and Irwin Goldstein, Pfizer had struck marketing gold. Partly thanks to Goldstein's insistence that sexual dysfunction was common and should be talked about, "erectile dysfunction" and "ED" entered layperson lingo. Impaired (male) performance in the bedroom went overnight from a shameful secret stashed in the basement to the slick penthouse of acceptability—and profitability. Other drug companies rushed to get FDA approval for ED medications, and today the pharmaceutical marketplace is crowded with numerous options for medical therapy to enhance and ensure that male virility can persist into senescence. Today an estimated thirty million men are affected by ED and twenty million American men have tried Viagra.[12]

Market Expansion

Once Viagra had achieved dominance over the market for men with ED, the Pfizer marketing geniuses expanded their target audience to healthy men. The new message was not "Viagra can fix your broken penis" but "Viagra can help you *enhance* and *optimize* your sex life."

The prescription target audience was far bigger now: men with ED *and* men without.

The new crop of ads for ED meds were also directed toward women. Ads showing men and women smiling at each other in a bathtub implied that if your male partner took Viagra, then loving and satisfying sex was sure to follow. DTC ads cautioned—and intrigued—viewers with the information that Viagra could cause a four-hour erection. Wink wink, what a terrible "side effect" for men wanting to have teenage erection capabilities in middle age. But did the smiling, relieved, and relaxed women in the ED commercials accurately represent female partners of American Viagra users? Were *they* enjoying their partners' newfound four-hour erections?

What About Us Women?

What *was* the effect on women of a seismically successful drug launch that became a cultural phenomenon? I asked my patients this question, from women who were there in the late 1990s when Viagra emerged, to women who are currently dating. In both cases, the women fall into three categories. For some, sharing their bedroom with Viagra allowed a return to the joy of penetrative sex and a resumption of coital sexual relations. "Once my husband got Viagra and he could have an erection again, it felt like the old days, and it has allowed us to revive some parts of our earlier sex life," one of my patients remarked.

Some couples, in contrast, simply learn to live with ED; for them, Viagra is unnecessary and unwanted. Says Sally, a retired science teacher, "We talked about it and decided that if Ned can't have an erection, then that is what his body is meant to do, or not do, and that taking a medication—which can have side effects—just to have a hard penis, is not necessary for us to enjoy being intimate. We are aging together, and we want to do so in a natural way."

A third group of women, probably the largest demographic, have an altogether different perspective. These are the women who have been sharing their stories, their frustrations, and their bewilderment with me for years; these are the women who inspired the writing of this book. These women suffer from what I call Viagravation. For them, Viagra is responsible for widening their own personal Bedroom Gap.

Perhaps it comes as no surprise that there is an unspoken awkwardness between men and women about lack of female sexual desire, lack of ability to lubricate, which is only exacerbated in the face of a middle-aged partner with a Viagra-primed penis. One patient described it "like a rocket" and another called it "frighteningly rigid, like a purple spear." These women are frustrated and annoyed that the Little Blue Pill for their partner has created a disconnect in their intimate lives. They feel like they are suddenly in a battle they cannot win. Their male partners are experiencing a sexual Renaissance while they are left to wither in the Middle Ages.

Armed with a diamond-shaped magic pill, my patients' partners seem to want sex more often, regularly, and repeatedly. The women are mostly peri- or postmenopausal and many have lost interest in sex, and when they do want it, and do have it, they feel betrayed by their anatomy's lack of responsiveness. Viagra was not designed with the natural aging of the female genitourinary system in mind. To be sure, the Little Blue Pill did not single-handedly cause the Bedroom Gap; men and women have always had different needs and desires and functions, sexually speaking. But the sexual tsunami of ED medications has left a mess in the bedrooms of baby boomers and now many Gen Xers.

Angie, age forty-five, is married to Clay, age forty-eight. She told me, "Ever since he got Cialis, Clay wants sex all the time! It's like he has to prove to himself that he can still do it like when he was in his twenties. I am afraid to cuddle with him at night because he takes that as an excuse to want to have sex. I just want to be able to kiss him or play footsie without us having to have sex. It's like the Cialis makes him horny."

Medications for ED don't directly make men "horny," but it is commonly known in sexual medicine circles that the brain circuitry from desire to arousal to sex for men is much straighter, simpler, and shorter than it is for women. So when a cuddle from Angie triggers a desire for sex in Clay, and he's got a performance guarantee from Cialis, he has little reason not to engage. If the apex of (heterosexual) male pleasure is vaginal penetration and ejaculation, then erection is a prerequisite for reaching the sexual summit. Viagra not only made erections happen, it made them stay harder and last longer. What does that math look like for a lot of men? More hard-ons plus longer lasting ones equal endless sexual summits.

Female Sexual Function Gets Medicalized Too

Yes, the story of Viagra is a story, at least in part, of the medicalization of male sexual function. While it is not a bad thing for men to want to improve or enhance erection, we have seen that it has widened the sexual gulf between men and their female partners. Viagra solved some problems but created others, and in general, women are on the receiving end of the problems it has caused. I have queried the couples who have sought my help over the years what role they believe Viagra or other ED drugs play in their sexual issues. While the women were well aware of the changes it has wrought, I find it interesting that very few men see ED medications as playing any role at all.

According to author Meika Loe, "The Viagra phenomenon has exposed the workings of male privilege on a global scale, making visible the power imbalances of gender in medical research, care, and coverage in America and beyond."[13] Loe points out that Viagra was approved and made available to men in Japan before the birth control pill was available to women(!).

The route to sexual satisfaction for women is different than that for men. For women, as New York sex therapist Esther Perel has put it, "Desire is often between the ears more than between the legs." Perel describes how women need a story; they want to be noticed, to be wooed, to have conversation, to make a connection, then have sex. Desire in their case is "contextual, subjective, layered on a lattice of emotion."[14] For men, sex is the connection, the language of intimacy and potentially of love. Female sexual function is more abstract, harder to describe, and harder to fix than simply firming up a limp penis.

Addyi, the First Female Sex Drug

The most prevalent sexual issue for midlife women is a lack of desire. So it is no wonder that the first medication to gain FDA approval for female sexual function was aimed at improving desire. Enter flibanserin.

Flibanserin, branded as Addyi but also known as "Pink Viagra," was the first FDA-approved drug to treat any type of female sexual dysfunction. Addyi was specifically created to treat women diagnosed with female hypoactive sexual desire disorder (HSDD).

HSDD is formally defined as "a deficiency or absence of sexual fantasies and desire for sexual activity. The disturbance must cause marked distress or interpersonal difficulty."[15] This specific definition, as it turned out, would cause marked distress for the drug's makers, as the FDA used it to set stringent standards for the drug's approval.

Like female sexuality as a whole, Addyi's mechanism of action has been described as unclear, but we actually know a lot about how it works.[16] Addyi is an oral pill taken every day that studies have shown improves sexually satisfying events by 0.5 to 1 per month. Yes, you heard that right. That's it. From 0.5 to 1. This means women who use it can expect between zero and one extra sexual experience per month. This is hardly packing a sexual punch.

Big Pharma company Boerhinger Ingelheim had spent roughly $900 million to develop and market Addyi, only to have it fail to gain FDA approval in June 2010 by a single vote of 10–1. The FDA claimed the drug was ineffective and that benefits to female sexual function were outweighed by side effects such as "loss of consciousness and depression."[17] This is ironic given that Addyi was first studied as an antidepressant. The company then tried and failed again in 2013. At that point, a tiny pharma company, Sprout, acquired the rights to Addyi, mounted an extensive advocacy campaign that included appeals to women's rights groups, and, two years later, in August 2015, the FDA finally approved Addyi.[18] Women cheered and celebrated. Finally, finally, something for *us*.

But Addyi's approval was met with mixed reviews and accompanied by a bioethical mess. On the one hand, efforts to get FDA sanction for a drug for female sexual dysfunction had come to fruition—we finally had a tool in the sexual toolkit for women. On the other hand, we had to creatively push and persistently pressure through advocacy groups such as Even the Score, which lobbied for Addyi's approval. The problem, according to a bioethics research institute called the Hastings Center, is that Even the Score was created and supported by Sprout pharmaceuticals itself, which hired feminist speakers and recruited and paid consumer advocacy groups to pressure the FDA. Hastings felt that using women's advocacy groups was unethical and discredited both the validity of the data submitted and the drug approval process. For its part, Even the Score used the approval challenges Addyi faced as evidence of an FDA mired in sexism.

The challenges continued. Just a few days after gaining FDA approval, Sprout was acquired by Valeant pharma for $1 billion. Apparently even female sex sells, or so thought executives at Valeant. But with such a wobbly launch, and such disappointing sales, Valeant soon sold the drug back to Sprout for a percentage of sales.

Addyi, on One Condition

Even when Addyi was finally approved by the FDA that summer of 2015 after the two prior failed attempts, its approval was conditional. Physicians and even pharmacists had to be "certified" to prescribe Addyi. The FDA wanted to be sure physicians understood that there were biological *and* psychological causes for lack of desire in women. In their view, Addyi should be prescribed to women who demonstrated *six months or longer of persistent lack of sexual desire* that caused *marked distress*. No Addyi for the woman who was just having a low patch in her marriage or a stressful time at work.

And, although Addyi had been shown to be safe and effective at increasing sexual desire and sexually satisfying events in both pre- and postmenopausal women, it was only approved for premenopausal women, which means it wasn't covered by insurance if you were postmenopausal.[19] If that isn't the perfect example of intersectional sexism and ageism, I don't know what is. We, the patriarchal FDA, care about you and your desire for sex as long as you are young enough to have a vagina worth fucking. But once you get past menopause, if you don't want sex, we don't want you.

In 2019 the FDA finally removed the certification mandate for physicians and pharmacists. Sprout pharmaceuticals had planned a big marketing campaign around a now-easier-to-prescribe Addyi for early 2020. Sadly this coincided with the explosion of the COVID pandemic, and Addyi's exciting new launch was drowned out by more pressing health care issues. Even without the COVID complications, the damage had already been done; physicians felt the drug was labor intensive to prescribe. In truth, Addyi is no more dangerous than the antidepressants that physicians in the United States prescribe at the drop of a hat. Why then did the FDA make this drug so damn hard for physicians to offer their patients? Here we see yet another example of a real and clear double standard with respect to FDA-imposed hurdles in the name of safety for a drug to improve female sexual desire.

Viagra sold a billion dollars in its first year and instantly became a household name, while Addyi has poor insurance coverage, middling clinical results, and sputtered both on arrival and relaunch. Viagra has widespread insurance coverage, is available through clinician prescription, and is sold directly to consumers via successful internet sites such as Roman. It is well marketed, widely available, and an absolute boon to the midlife male sexual experience.

So what about the women who want to have sex? Can they keep pace with their Viagra-popping partners? Not likely. Is there a "Viagra" for them?

Is There a "Female Viagra?"

If Addyi was created to increase desire in women, what about something aimed more at the clitoris—something to promote clitoral stimulation, akin to the Viagra effect on the penis? Is there such a thing as a female Viagra?

Viagra has been studied in women but found to have little to no positive effect on sexual function. Kim Catrall took Viagra in a *Sex and the City* episode and became super amped up for sex, but that's

Hollywood. In real life Viagra only indirectly improves libido in men by improving their erectile potential. For women, the desire for and ability to have satisfying sex is more nuanced, more complex, and not really dependent on clitoral erection.

Testosterone for Women: The Path to Intrinsa

The hunt for a female Viagra has proved challenging. As Pfizer and other pharma companies poured money into research teams to study Viagra and biosimilars for effectiveness in women, the urologist and researcher Irwin Goldstein and others began to explore testosterone use for women. Proctor and Gamble (P&G) spent many millions in the 1990s to develop and market the first testosterone patch for women, called Intrinsa.

This seemed like good news. As already mentioned, most respected thought leaders in women's health now agree that replacing some of the lost testosterone after menopause is one way to help women's sexual health.[20] And P&G's testosterone patch had potential. According to menopause expert Dr. James Simon, a past president of the North American Menopause Society, "The [testosterone] patch came very close to getting approval, but the FDA rejected it by one vote. This was the closest we came in the US to having a safe and effective source of testosterone replacement for women."[21] And so the hunt for female Viagra continued.

Vyleesi, Female Viagra 2.0

The second drug to be FDA-approved for female sexual function after Addyi was bremelanotide, sold as Vyleesi, which was formulated as an on-demand injection. Yes—you heard that correctly. Vyleesi is an injection you give yourself (the needle is tiny and actually painless) an hour or so before you (don't) want to have sex, so you will want to have sex.

Palatin Technologies launched Vyleesi in 2019. It activates several receptors in the brain, but its exact mechanism of improving female desire is a bit of a mystery. Its most bothersome side effect, which does decrease with each subsequent injection, is nausea and vomiting. Throwing up isn't most women's idea of how to get in the mood for sex. In Chapter 7 we'll learn about what it's like to use Vyleesi and discuss some hacks for a good experience.

Women Still Left Wanting

The bottom line is that the development, marketing, commercial and cultural success of medications for erectile dysfunction such as Viagra, when compared with the lack of effective and available medical therapies for female sexual issues, underscore some important (and sometimes depressing) points.

First, we are living in an age of medicalization/pathologization of normal human aging, including sexual function. On the one hand, the medicalization of sex is a good thing—it has reduced the sense of shame surrounding sex as a topic. Pfizer's efforts to bring awareness of the pervasiveness of ED and other similar issues into our homes and our doctor's exam rooms has certainly led to more open dialogue about sexual issues, especially male-centered ones.

But the upsides of sexual medicalization don't seem to be working for both genders: Prevailing androcentrism and the glorification of the sexually amped up alpha male in modern-day society remains troubling, and the prioritization of male pleasure over female pleasure stubbornly persists. Medicalizing female desire may trivialize its complexities and nuances. As clinical psychologist Sheryl Kingsberg writes, "How a woman responds to sexual cues is highly dependent on a number of distinct, yet related, factors. Researchers have attempted to explain the female sexual response for decades, but no single model reigns supreme. Proper female sexual function relies on the interplay of somatic, psychosocial and neurobiological factors; misregulation of any of these components could result in sexual dysfunction."[22]

Relational, cultural, consent, reproductive, and even religious factors are at play for women as we navigate sexual choices and wrestle with changes in desire and pleasure as we age. Since the biopharma community has supercharged the male sexual world with medical treatment options while largely neglecting female sexual issues, women must look inward for help. Part 2 of this book looks at closing the Bedroom Gap from within our own bedrooms. We'll explore female sexual desire, then pleasure, and finish with (sorry, I couldn't help myself!) orgasms; first let's take a look at the particularities of sex today, and why the societal permeation of porn, saturation of social media, and digital dating bring both benefits and challenges to our sexual relationships.

Chapter 3

Sex Today

Think back to your own initiation into sex. What did you really know about sex? We arrive at our first sexual experience supposedly already knowing "how to do it." We don't dare admit we are not really sure how to give a blow job, what sounds to make, whether to keep our eyes open or closed, how to know for sure if we had an orgasm, if we should use lube much less which one, whether we should clean ourselves before or after sex, or both. The media images of sex we learn from never include couples asking "What do you like? How could I do better? Do you mind if we try it differently next time?" Those bits of (important) dialogue do not make the director's cut. Since much of what we learn about sex is from watching, listening to, and reading media, we begin our sex lives with the belief that it is normal to want to have sex, that it is important to be "good at" sex, and that sex is just performed correctly and well without discussion or dialogue about it. This chapter is about the pitfalls, pleasures, and challenges of sex today.

Sex and Intimacy in the Zoom Era

Many women today tell me they "don't have time" for sex. When I shared this observation with my uber-practical girlfriend Julie, she quipped, "What is the big deal? It takes ten minutes." Julie, you are on to something. Many couples I work with have a sexual routine with a predictable cuddle, kiss, lubricate, penetrate, and ejaculate series of events. Yeah, we have sex. Done.

What my patients mean, really, is that they don't have time for intimacy, for sexual play, conversation, experimentation, and fantasy, for roleplay and foreplay and afterplay and alone time. They don't have time for sexual connection. We as a society don't have the time and don't make the time for the foundational relational building blocks of a good sex life. We expect sex to fit neatly into a slot in our day, somewhere between Zoom calls, the grocery store, and Netflix. To destroy any hope of making time for meaningful, pleasure-focused sex, we often bring at least one or two addictive, interactive devices to bed with us, and unfortunately, I don't mean vibrators.

Where's My Phone?

It is nearly impossible to keep our phones out of the bedroom. Over 70 percent of Americans who own smartphones take them to bed with them.[1] To make matters so much worse, 35 percent of people check their phones immediately after sex, and 10 percent check their smartphone *during* sex.[2] (My money says this is an underreported phenomenon and the actual numbers are far worse.) No wonder it is so hard to be in the moment! Don't kid yourself that charging the phone on a nightstand or end table in your bedroom means you don't have it with you. If you can see it, or hear the dings, beeps, and chimes, or just see the glow change with a new notification, you are still tethered to its addictive grasp. If you want to de-stress your life and improve your sex life, charge your phone overnight in another room—so you can recharge too.

The Digital Dating Age

Technology has permeated every aspect of our lives, including sex and dating. When my friend Frank and his wife, Mindy, separated in their mid-forties, they both began using dating apps. Frank, educated, successful, athletic, and interesting, shared that soon after creating his profile, he was going out on five dates per week, and between two and three of those dates converted into a sexual encounter. Eventually the fun and pleasure of easily obtainable sex wore off, and Frank wanted to find a long-term companion.

"At first, I was like a kid in a candy factory," he told me. "But after a while, it became so easy to find women to date, that they all started to blur together, and I decided I needed a system. If they didn't rate at least 7 out of 10 on our first date, I didn't date them again, even if they wanted to or just wanted to have sex."

Mindy had a different experience. Whereas Frank was finding matches with women of any age range, Mindy found age-related constraints to her ability to match. "All the men my age wanted to date younger women, often women who were still open to having children; I was forty-six and had four teenage kids, so I was off the radar for many men my age. I got plenty of interest from the sixty-to-seventy-year-olds looking for a 'younger woman,' but these were not men I could see myself with twenty years from now. I wanted someone who was fun to be with but also someone to grow old with. Most of the younger men in their thirties (and even twenties!) were looking for casual sex. I went on a bit of a sex spree right when we separated, I think out of anger and revenge for his affair, and to prove to myself that I was fuckable. It felt good to meet other men and have sex in different ways. We had been married for over twenty years!"

Online dating is now the most common way to meet potential sex partners. According to a Pew Research study, one in ten partnered adults in the United States met their partner on a dating app.[3] In 2018 there were forty million Americans using dating apps; by 2028 that number is expected to reach sixty-five million users. Nearly 80 percent of the under-thirty crowd uses online dating apps, and one in six Americans over fifty have used them.[4] Tinder is the most widely used dating app today across all ages, but in the over-fifty cohort, Match .com reigns supreme, though eHarmony and other sites are also popular. All different kinds of dating apps abound, and you can find one that works in the way that you like.[5]

To Have (Sex) and Have Not: The Sexless Marriage

Most couples have sex about once a week in the first decade after marriage (fifty-eight times a year specifically, on average), after which the frequency decreases. Couples in their twenties have sex about eighty times per year. By age forty-five, the frequency is about sixty times per year, and by age sixty-five, it drops to about twenty times per year.[6] Put another way, the percentage of adults having *weekly sex* drops with each decade of aging from 44 percent (adults age 40–49), to 34 percent (age 50–59) to 25 percent (age 60–69) to 16 percent (age 70 and over).[7] Yes, it's a drop-off, but it does mean that one third of couples in their fifties have sex once a week, and one in six couples is still having sex once a week over age seventy. Not bad! Three studies looking at a total of over thirty thousand people found there was a relationship between sexual frequency and happiness, but only to a point. Sex more than once a week did not lead to more happiness in the study participants.[8] (Yes, you can tell your husband this right away, and no, you are not abnormal because you don't have sex four times a week like your friends—supposedly—do.) But what about couples who have stopped having sex altogether?

Psychologist and author Esther Perel reminds us that "we . . . live in an age of entitlement; personal fulfillment, we believe, is our due. In the West, sex is a right linked to our individuality, our self-actualization, and our freedom. Thus, most of us now arrive at the altar after years of sexual nomadism. By the time we tie the knot, we've hooked up, dated, cohabited, and broken up. We used to get married and have sex for the first time. Now we get married and stop having sex with others. Sometimes, we get married and stop having sex with each other."[9]

A Sexual Spark to Try at Home

Fixing the enormous sexual gulf in a sexless marriage is no easy task; it requires vulnerability, openness, and honesty. But there is a simple starting point. Try taking some nonsexual first steps: spending time together, talking with each other, being present in each other's lives. This is, for many women (and men as well) a turn on in and of itself. Later in the book I talk about "G-rated masturbation," touching yourself in a non-genitally focused way as a way to build self-interest in sex. Well, it is the same for partnered sex. Not interested? Not attracted anymore? Not feeling sexy or sexual yourself? Try nonsexual, non-genital touching. Rubbing shoulders, feeling arm muscles. Go for a walk and hold hands. Wash his or her hair. Give a back rub. A foot massage. Even just nibble an earlobe. Sometimes the smallest actions or sensations can spark arousal and interest.

My patient Courtney, forty years old, attractive, and energetic, came to see me once and started in right away with her concerns: "I am really happy, and I'm healthy. I have no medical problems. We've been married twelve years and Raj, my husband, is my best friend. Our life is great. Our house is perfect. Our two girls are amazing. But we haven't had sex in a really long time. And I think it is affecting our marriage." She paused, inhaled. "My husband, well, he is not happy about it," she said. Twenty percent of couples, including Courtney and Raj, are living in a "sexless marriage," defined objectively as sex less than ten times per year, or no sex for a year, or subjectively defined as a marriage in which one or both members of the couple are unhappy with the frequency of sex.[10] People who live in sexless marriages report feeling "frustrated, unloved, undesirable, unattractive and lonely."[11] We know that loneliness has negative health consequences, including heart attacks, strokes, cancers, eating disorders, drug abuse, sleep deprivation, depression, alcoholism, and anxiety, as well as acceleration of Alzheimer's and cognitive decline.[12] How did Courtney and Raj, who seem to have so much to connect them, get here?

In a 2016 TED talk, sex therapist Maureen McGrath noted that sex is controlled by the partner with the low desire.[13] Often the sex-starved partner broaches the subject, at first delicately or sometimes as a direct request for sex. Stating a sexual want requires some courage and vulnerability. When the request is rejected—"Not tonight. I have a headache. I'm tired. I want to watch this show."— that vulnerability is replaced by contempt and anger, says McGrath, which in turn can lead to sexual withdrawal. This can lead to infidelity and even divorce. Remember that rejection hurts. Be very careful of rejecting sexual requests, especially again and again. This is a warning sign that the relationship is anemic and in need of an attention transfusion as much as a sexual one. McGrath puts it this way: "Sex is the barometer of the state of affairs of a marriage." Without it, even strong marriages can sometimes go awry. A sexless marriage may be a result of aging and a mutual decision not to have sex, but it can also be a product of, or a prelude to, infidelity.

Infidelity

Let's be honest—infidelity has been around as long as sex and human bonding; it is universal, ubiquitous, and thanks to the anonymity of dating apps, the barrier to entry may now be easier. Affairs are a tricky thing, and since cheating peaks for both sexes around midlife, it is worth talking about it.

Why does infidelity happen? Sometimes it is a by-product of a sexless marriage, but sometimes infidelity occurs in a relationship in which one or both people are feeling unsatisfied with their sex life, for whatever reason. A common reason for infidelity in both sexes is a desire for *novelty*, good ol' dopamine catching up with us. Men reported that a big motivator for infidelity was *sexual* dissatisfaction—namely, they had an interest in specific novel sexual acts such as anal sex that their partner didn't share.

Women, on the other hand, most frequently reported *relationship* dissatisfaction as a driver to seek another relationship, particularly when they feel unappreciated.[14] But even couples who describe a happy, high-functioning relationship experience infidelity. I have often felt, having listened to many of my patients share their stories of relationship infidelity, that an affair sometimes has less to do with the shortcomings of the (betrayed) partner than with the adulterer's realization of his/her own shortcomings and a need for something to compliment or fulfill or make up for them. It is about where one is in one's own life, and about needing and seeking change, perhaps in tempo with one's own evolution as an adult.

Esther Perel examined the "why" of infidelity in an article she penned for *The Atlantic* in 2017, addressing the conundrum of "why do happily married couples cheat?" "Sometimes when we seek the gaze of another," Perel writes, "it's not our partner we are turning away from, but the person we have become. We are not looking for another lover so much as another version of ourselves." She continues, "So often, the most intoxicating 'other' that people discover in an affair is not a new partner; it's a new self."[15] This may explain why 25 percent of Tinder users are in a committed relationship![16] In looking online for a new version of a partner, they are looking for a new version of themselves.

Another reason for infidelity is to satisfy unmet expectations. This is part and parcel of the Bedroom Gap itself: We expect our partner to remain sexually vibrant, orgasmically capable, perpetually curious. But bodies age, desires and wants change, capacity for orgasm or lubrication may diminish, people get bored, distracted, or just plain tired. Relationships need to evolve to stay fresh, and when they don't, especially if there is also poor communication, expectations go unmet and affairs can happen. Perel explains the enormity of the challenge of staying interested in and interesting to our life partner when she writes, "We expect a lot from one relationship. Never before have our expectations of marriage taken on such epic proportions. We still want everything the traditional family was meant to provide—security, respectability, property, and children—but now we also want our partner to love us, to desire us, to be *interested* in us. We should be best friends and trusted confidants, and passionate lovers to boot." This is a lot of roles to master for one partner!

Perel continues, "We want our chosen one to offer stability, safety, predictability, and dependability. And we want that very same person to supply awe, mystery, adventure, and risk. We expect comfort and edge, familiarity and novelty, continuity and surprise . . .

love will remain unconditional, intimacy enthralling, and sex oh so exciting, with one person, for the long haul. And the long haul keeps getting longer."[17] Here, Perel underscores that it is no easy task to stay sexually desirable, and to desire sex with one partner, for a large chunk of an increasingly long lifespan, and hence increasingly long sexspan.

Longer Lifespans, Longer Sexspans

Sexspan, according to urologist Dr. Mohit Khera, is the portion of your lifespan during which you have interest in and ability to engage in sex. Dr. Khera believes, as do I, that "sexual health is one of the best barometers of overall health" and that optimizing our sexspan has massive health benefits.

As humans increase their lifespan, their sexspan is also increasing. How long is longer? In a first-world country, women can expect to live on average eighty-two years and men seventy-seven.[18] In the least developed countries, these figures are sixty-seven and sixty-three years. Due to career aspirations, the average age of marriage in developed countries has increased and is currently around age twenty-eight for women and thirty and a half for men.[19] We may end up living a half century under the same roof with the same person and the same marital and sexual expectations! This is a long time to be satisfied, sexually and otherwise, with one person.

Sexual dysfunction, Khera notes, is "a couple's disease," because if one partner has sexual dysfunction, it nearly always affects the other partner. His three tips for optimizing sexspan include: (1) Focus on the four pillars of health (sleep, diet, exercise, and social connection) for yourself; (2) Focus on your partner's health (the same four pillars of health) and your partner's engagement in sex; and (3) Understand hormones, especially testosterone.[20]

Know Thy Hormones, and Those of Thy Partner

Testosterone levels for men normally peak around age eighteen, then drop as men age. Up to 39 percent of men over forty-five have low testosterone, defined as under 300 ng/dl by the American Urological Association (AUA), which sets a normal range of testosterone for men at 450–600 mg/dl. Men with symptomatic low testosterone levels can opt for treatment with TRT, testosterone replacement therapy. TRT comes in many forms, from an intranasal gel to topical gels to pellets to an injection or a patch, all standardized and FDA-approved. TRT is the male version of HT, which consists of estrogen and progesterone, the hormone therapy we (far too infrequently) offer to women.

Unfortunately, the medical powers that be seem to have forgotten that *women also make testosterone* (over three times as much testosterone as estrogen in fact) and that women also become *testosterone deficient with age*. We don't really know the percentage of women with low testosterone because, sadly, it hasn't yet been considered as a menopausal or health metric for women. And yet, the symptoms of low "T" in men—low energy, low mood, low libido, increased fat deposition—mirror many of the symptoms of menopause in women. Gee, could it be that women with low testosterone have some of the same symptoms as men with low testosterone?

What's more, men found to have low testosterone also have elevated rates of diabetes, heart attack, osteoporosis, and depression, conditions that also develop in postmenopausal women.[21] Menopause hormone therapy should include replacement of testosterone as well as estrogen and progesterone as a way not only to boost libido, which we do for men, but also to improve women's overall health and lifespan. (I mean, is it just me or is this kind of a no-brainer?) In the United States today, only about 3 percent of women who could benefit from short- and long-term effects of hormone therapy are using it.

The Gendered Cheating Gap

Is it normal to slip on a wedding band and speak some vows and then not have sexual interest in others, not be sexually curious, not want to eat any cereal other than Cheerios for the next fifty years? I think most of us stay sexually curious, aware of the sexuality of the gender we are attracted to, but become ring-and-vow-prohibited from exploring that curiosity. Perel finds this concept a touch unrealistic as well: "Our desire for others is supposed to miraculously evaporate, vanquished by the power of this singular attraction." Interest in others doesn't disappear—in fact, it increases over time. There is a gendered cheating gap that widens with age; in their twenties and thirties, men and women cheat equally, but in their forties, the percentage of men who cheat rises more than the percentage of women who cheat. This trend continues even into people's seventies and eighties.[22]

The gender cheating gap is wider among older adults

% who reported having sex with someone other than spouse while married

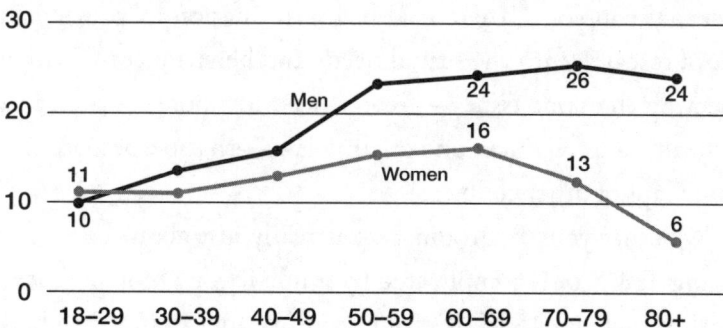

Based on adults who are either currently married or have been married before.
Source: General Social Survey 2010–2016

The sharpest increase in the rate of infidelity for men is between ages fifty and fifty-nine. Hmm. Might there be a hormonal/

menopausal basis for this? The most common age for women to see me for help with painful sex and loss of libido is in their mid-to-late fifties. Coincidence? I think not. There is about a five-year lag between when the ovaries cease to produce estrogen and testosterone (the average age of menopause is 51.5) and when women stream into my office stating that it feels like sandpaper, or a cactus, or shards of glass are in their vagina, and either they never want to have sex again or they want this surprise nightmare fixed. It's no wonder these hormonally anemic female fifty-somethings become averse to sex and are not what their partners signed up for when they got married twenty or thirty years earlier.

The gendered cheating gap even persists in couples with open relationships. About 4 percent of couples in the United States participate in consensual or ethical nonmonogamy (CNM or ENM, two interchangeable terms) where both partners consent to relationships outside the primary relationship. Among CNM couples there is more participation among straight men than straight women, and more participation among bisexual and gay/lesbian couples than heterosexual couples.[23] There is also discrimination by providers and a lack of research into the sexual needs and behaviors of CNM adults, reflecting the same issues—greater need for more research into sexual health and reeducations of clinicians—that perpetuate the Bedroom Gaps of other couples.

Whether your Bedroom Gap is really just about being tired, or lacking desire, or is complicated by infidelity or a more nuanced relationship such as CNM, it's important to understand the challenges of being sexually active today, where most women with low libido and sexual pain lack access to information, and treatment and other willing sex partners are sometimes just a click away.

PART TWO

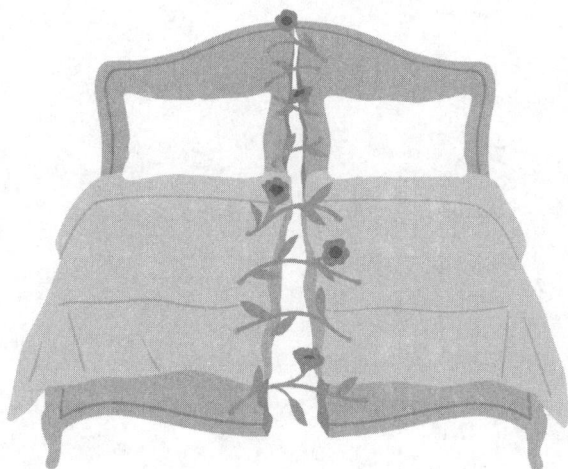

Chapter 4

Desire

Gender equality, and dare I say it, freedom and power in society, may be measured by our ability to acknowledge that everyone deserves sexual pleasure and that both men and women feel—and deserve to feel—desire.

But that's not how it looked for women back in the day, and not for women in our present society either. Boys are taught that desire is natural, that sexual dreams, fantasies, and penetrative sex are the norm, that masturbation is fine from cradle to grave, that men have "needs." Men with robust sexual appetites—desire—are admired as an archetype of their gender; women with robust sexual appetites are either reviled as "slutty" or simply not understood.

Girls are taught about menstruation, but that's where sex ed gets stuck for us. We are loath to admit that "good girls" touch themselves or talk about—much less desire—sexual pleasure. We are taught not to masturbate, or at least to be ashamed if we do. Even if we're not embarrassed about it, we definitely shouldn't *talk* about masturbation. On the one hand, we are taught that our bodies are for reproduction; on the other, we are told we should try not to get pregnant, at least not until we are supposed to get pregnant.

When and if we are allowed to have sex, we are taught to have sex when and how a man wants to have sex with us. We are not taught to have agency over our body, our sexual preferences, our own desire, our own capacity for pleasure. This sociocultural minimization of female pleasure in human sexuality has persisted over millennia. It's a sexual double standard that is at the core of the Bedroom Gap. We have been taught, in a thousand different ways, that we are not meant to be actively owning decisions around sex.

Don't Women in Midlife Care About Sex?

Actually, they do. And they don't. Lack of sexual desire is the most common form of sexual dysfunction in women of all age groups, with about 10 percent reporting distress as a result of their lack of desire.[1] When we look at some of the factors, it all makes sense. Many of us have spent the better parts of our lives in a rather predictable role: mother, wife, coworker, daughter, sister, friend. Up until our fifties, we might spend our lives focused on achieving, becoming, nurturing (and that includes having sex *for* our partner's pleasure rather than our own). But our fifties are often a time for reflecting on what *we* want. To "give fewer f—ks" about anyone and anything, as some women say. That includes sex on our terms, with or without a partner, with or without orgasm, frequently or rarely or never.

For some of us, it means freeing ourselves from the feeling of "I have to" and deciding to remove sex from our relationship. We may become asexual or just enjoy masturbation. Or we may just morph sex into cuddling or oral sex or just no penis-in-vagina (PIV) sex. For some couples, this is mutually agreed upon and works fine. For others, it's a source of strife. Of course, removal of sex from a relationship is not just a source of strife for men, but for women too. Some women who are wanting to *want* sex are frustrated by their lack of desire. For still others, the end of family responsibilities as kids move out, paired with the end of period issues and contraceptive concerns, is liberating. They experience a sexual renaissance of sorts, wanting to explore and grow with their partner or with new partners.

Meanwhile, the sexual wellness market is booming, and some women in midlife are embracing the many new options out there for toys, lube, even libido-enhancing gummies. Smart vibrators that give feedback on orgasm are here—more on this later![2] Apps with erotic stories abound, finally written by and for a female audience.[3] It is a great time to be a woman looking to expand her sexual horizons, even within the boundaries of a marriage.

So if you are interested in getting more interested in sex, or want to have better sex, good news abounds. Let's start with the best news, so you can stop worrying so much. You don't have to have a raging or even modest libido to have satisfying sex. I know, I can imagine your skepticism but hear me out.

Every day at my clinic, women tell me, "I have zero libido. I don't care if I ever have sex again." Then they continue, "But I feel bad for my partner and it's affecting our relationship and our sex life. So I need to find my libido again. I want to *want* to have sex, and I don't."

That's when I get to explain the bombshell news: Good sexual experience doesn't always start with sexual desire. This seems almost nonsensical, but it's true. Traditional sex models tell us that desire begets arousal, which then leads to sex. But haven't we learned by now that nothing is that simple when it comes to these matters?

Sexual desire is complex. It is at its core psychological: an emotional state rather than a physical state, a subjective feeling that can be triggered and developed through imagination and fantasies.

Arousal, on the other hand, is purely physical. It's the physiologic response to stimuli—the dilation of blood vessels, the rush of color, the seeping of lubricating fluid, the erection of a penis.

Desire has been considered a distinct phase of sexual response, a necessary prerequisite to arousal and orgasm, but this may be an oversimplification. Another way to look at desire is that it is something that can develop before *or* after arousal, and that it can persist through arousal and climax. So which comes first, desire or arousal?

Spontaneous Versus Receptive Desire

The answer, like sex itself, is complex and nuanced. *It depends.* There are two types of sexual desire: spontaneous desire and receptive desire. Spontaneous desire, as the name implies, is desire that comes over you when you're watching a video of a steamy sex scene or checking out the super fit person with fine features next to you in line at the supermarket. Spontaneous desire happens whether you were born with a penis or vagina, identify as male or female, or are gender fluid, but it seems to occur more readily in those born with a Y chromosome and a penis.[4]

Receptive desire, on the other hand, occurs more commonly in biological females. Receptive desire, based on the research of Dr. Rosemary Basson, a professor of psychiatry who studies human sexual response, refers to *desire that develops as a response to sexual arousal.* It flips around the whole desire-first, arousal-second script. This is information that should make you feel relieved of the burden that you have to "find or regain desire" to jump-start your sex life. It bears repeating: Receptive desire, which is your likely flavor of choice, develops *after* some level of arousal, not before.

Research by the renowned Kinsey Institute supports Basson's theory that sexual desire can be cultivated, or developed as a response to sexual arousal. Said another way, it does *not* need to be initially present for a satisfying sexual encounter. So ladies, give yourself grace! *You don't have to have substantial or even modest baseline sexual desire to have gratifying sex.* You can be kissing, caressing, just fooling around or doing some late-night cuddling and become aroused. Hopefully your partner can as well, and if so, as your nuzzling becomes more erotic in nature, sexual desire can be a quiet seed that germinates and flowers.

The Mind-Genital Connection

Another reason your libido might not be where you want it? The mind-genital connection. Ever feel like your mind is "in the mood" but your genitals aren't answering the call? Or maybe it's your mind that isn't in the game. Your partner lightly strokes your leg while you watch TV, and you can feel your genitals respond, but it's late, you're tired. Your brain is not on board.

These are two sides of the same coin, and there's actually a name for this: Arousal Non-Concordance. It is when physiological arousal and mental arousal are not happening at the same time. And it's common! Men experience this up to 50 percent of the time. It might seem like they are always on board for sex, but believe it or not, they also need to have both their head and their hard-on in the game at the same time. For women, that number is up to 90 percent, meaning only about 10 percent of the time is a woman mentally and physically in sync for sex.[5] Now can you see why it's so challenging to have *both* desire and arousal in *both* partners at the same time? Of course, it's not a given that you and your partner are always ready for sex!

How does this news make you feel? Liberated, I hope. Which should help put you in the right frame of mind for the next conversation we need to have. First, let's look at the factors that cause low desire, and second, let's show you how to get your mojo back.

What Causes Low Sexual Desire?

Our sexual experience has biological, psychological, and social determinants. We call this the biopsychosocial model of sex. Low desire can be caused by biological, personal, societal, educational, and even cultural causes. Let's look into some of the more common ones that might be affecting your own lack of desire.

Here are **seven causes of low sexual desire** that top the list:

1. Sexual pain
2. Sex education
3. Depression
4. Stress
5. Body image
6. Sexual inhibition
7. Attention (or lack of attention)

Let's look more deeply into this list, starting with sexual pain.

Sexual Pain: If Sex Hurts, We Don't Want to Do It

Sexual pain itself has many causes, but let's focus on ten in all, some of the most common and also some that often go undiagnosed.

1. Sexual Pain from GSM
GSM, or as it is more commonly known, vaginal atrophy, is a common culprit of sexual pain. It is a direct result of a lack of estrogen. But it is not the only gynecological issue that can result in painful sex.

2. Sexual Pain from Vulvodynia
Vulvodynia, simply put, is chronic vulvar pain without an identifiable cause. The most common symptoms of this underdiagnosed and underappreciated cause for sexual pain are burning, stinging, irritation, and a raw feeling.

*Vestibulo*dynia is vulvodynia at the opening to the vagina. Provoked vestibulodynia (PVD) is pain that occurs when the vestibule is touched or pressed—think speculum, tampon, vibrator, penis—or even from prolonged sitting or wearing tight pants. Vulvodynia can be idiopathic (no cause) or be hormonally mediated. We see the latter in some women who use birth control pills.

3. Sexual Pain and "The Pill"
Most birth control pills contain a form of estrogen and progesterone and can cause sexual pain by lowering testosterone and increasing a protein called SHBG that binds to testosterone and makes for less lubrication at the vestibule.[6]

4. Sexual Pain from Endometriosis
Sexual pain associated with endometriosis is usually felt deeper inside the body, triggered by deep thrusting. Endometriosis—a common condition in which the endometrial cells lining the uterus grow outside the uterus—can cause pain and infertility, and even after menopause, the scarring from endometriosis can lead to painful sex.[7]

5. Sexual Pain from Fibroids
Between 70 and 80 percent of women have fibroids—benign masses made of smooth muscle cells—that can range in size from a small pea to a melon. They can be asymptomatic or cause tremendous discomfort with sex. Sexual pain related to fibroids is usually positional and experienced with deep penetration or thrusting.

6. Sexual Pain from Surgical Scarring
Even if your fibroids or endometriosis have been surgically removed, you can have painful sex from scarring as your body heals from intra-abdominal surgery. Scarring, whether from a c-section, hysterectomy, or other procedures, can render internal organs immobile, even frozen in place, which can cause pain with sex.

7. Sexual Pain from Episiotomy
The pain from a vaginal delivery isn't always temporary. Episiotomies repaired incorrectly can make initial penetration a teeth-gritting experience decades after childbirth.

8. Sexual Pain from Cosmetic Gynecologic Surgery
Labiaplasty, the trimming of the size and shape of the labia minora for cosmetic purposes, has come into fashion lately, largely driven by the labia-free representation of female anatomy among porn stars. The vast majority of women, a whopping 87 percent, seek labiaplasty for visual and aesthetic reasons.[8]

9. Sexual Pain from Transgender Surgery
Another elective surgery that often results in sexual pain is the construction of a neovagina for a transwoman. These "vaginas" are technically functional but less expandable than a vagina in a woman who was born with one. More on this in Chapter 10.

10. Sexual Pain from Anti-Estrogen Medications and Radiation Therapy

Surgery isn't the only doctor-caused reason for sexual pain. Breast cancer survivors—and there are four million of them in the United States alone—frequently take anti-estrogen medications to reduce cancer recurrence. But these medications can have devastating sexual side effects, sapping the body of estrogen and causing an accelerated and severe version of GSM. Radiation therapy for cervical and uterine cancer can render the vagina a tube of stiff whitish tissue whose former elasticity and moisture is nearly impossible to restore. Sexual pain is an obvious reason for lack of desire, but your sexual education and the messages you learned about sex growing up impact your ideas about desire as well.

Sex Ed: Who Taught You That?!

Your relationship with sexual desire can be affected by something as simple and basic as how you were taught about sex growing up. When did these lessons happen in your life? Who was responsible for your education?

One of my good friends was raised in Ireland and attended a religion-based school, which reinforced what was intuited at home and in her community: that virginity was to be guarded like a treasure, that masturbation was a crime worse than murder (this was verbatim from her teachers), and that sex was a wifely duty, to be endured no matter the pain, because men have "needs." This was the 1970s and '80s. What we learn about sex and where we learn it matters. It impacts our lifelong approach to sex and desire. Despite the Bedroom Gap–inciting messages my friend was fed in school in Ireland, one study from the United Kingdom concluded that we feel less distress around sex when most of our education takes place in a school setting.[9] We will learn more about how good and early sex ed makes for fewer sexual problems in midlife in the next few chapters.

Depression, Happiness, and Sex

Even if you didn't get the message as a teenager that wanting sex was bad and wrong, there are plenty of other reasons you might not feel much desire as a big girl. Depression, for example, is strongly correlated with lack of sexual desire. In fact, it nearly doubles your chances of low sexual desire. Fifty percent of women with depression have low sexual desire, and sexual dysfunction of some type is seen in up to 75 percent of people with major depression.[10]

There is also a correlation between the frequency of sexual activity and happiness. (No, your partner did not pay me to write this. It's true!) Studies show that the happiest sexually active couples have sex weekly and that overall sexual well-being is closely related to general happiness.[11]

Stress and Sexual Desire

Depression is only one of the mood-related disorders that affects sexual well-being—stress is another major culprit. Modern society is stressed out. We are a multitasking, minute-by-minute scheduled, striving, smartphone-gripped culture. Being digitally addled and addicted to our screens is a recipe for sexual disaster. Optimizing every second of our lives for time and task has turned our days into frenzied, frenetic productivity orgies.

No wonder we never feel mentally free from our responsibilities. We're rarely fully present and our minds are almost never clear—two necessary criteria for actually enjoying sex. Our brains categorize intimacy and foreplay as "not productive." They don't fit naturally into a day of Zoom meetings, errands, and household to-dos. So we don't prioritize them. Even if we do manage to make time, chronic stress is well known to affect sexual dysfunction; it increases distract-ibility, intensifies pain with sex, and reduces genital sexual response, among other things—which we will discuss in more scientific detail in the next chapter![12]

Body Image

Our image of our own body can be a big source for low sexual desire. If you really aren't happy with your body, you really don't want to share that body, naked no less, with another person. Hack: The best time to push away distractions and make an honest and hopefully supportive assessment of your body is while bathing.

Getting Comfortable

Now that we've discussed all the reasons sexual desire might be lacking at this stage in our lives—for physical reasons and for emotional ones—let's start figuring out ways to tackle some of our concerns and get more comfortable with our relationship with sex.

The most important way I tell my patients to start to get comfortable with themselves and their desires (or lack thereof) is by getting to know themselves better. How? By taking a closer look at themselves—literally. It's time to get a little more intimate with the mirror. Get a makeup mirror (on a stand or handheld) and place it on the bathroom floor. Yes, I am going there. Many women are uncomfortable with their genital anatomy. Don't know what you're looking at? Can't name the parts? Totally normal. Let's have a look together.

First things first: Let's learn some new words. We often call all of it the vagina, but the vagina is just the inside. The outside is collectively called the vulva. Not the reliable Swedish car. Vulva. V-U-L-V-A. Five letters. Remember it for Wordle.

Use two fingers to gently separate the lips. The opening from the vulva into the vagina is called the vestibule, which is where a lot of women start to feel pain as they age. As we've discussed, the vestibule is very sensitive to changes in hormones. Postpartum or postmeno-pause (or even just from birth control pills, remember vulvodynia?), the vestibule (and its owner) suffers intensely from estrogen and/or testosterone deficiency. Sensitivity in the vestibule is what causes much of the discomfort with sex as we age.

The lips, or labia, come in two pairs. The labia majora, or bigger, outer lips, are more lateral. These are wide and puffy in youth but get saggy and deflated as we age. (Again, this is normal!) The thinner, more medial lips, or labia minora, are often asymmetrical and even different sized from each other (unless you're a porn star, in which case they've probably been surgically trimmed to near nonexistence). When patients want cosmetic labiaplasty, it's the labia minora that they want trimmed or evened out, or mostly removed. Sometimes they actually are entirely gone from the picture.

The urethral opening—the entrance to the urethra, the tube allowing the bladder to drain to the outside world—is actually in the vagina. It's a tiny, slit-like opening right at the upper/top vaginal wall just south of the clitoris.

You might know where to find your clitoris (if not, you will soon!), but you definitely wouldn't recognize a free-standing clitoris if it was walking down the street. Why? Because it's nearly all inter-nal. So, while you are checking yourself out down there, just remem-ber that the clitoris is just like a giant iceberg—only a small bit of it is above the water! Only the tip of the clitoris is visible on the outside of our bodies, but that tip, protected by a hood of tissue, is concentrated, supercharged erectile tissue, and a powerful source of female pleasure, just like a penis is for men.

In fact, the two have far more in common than you might've previously thought. Our labia majora are just our version of a scrotum. The slender, softer, non–hair bearing labia minora become the smooth inner surface of the penis, which hosts the urethra. And the penis itself, the star of the male genital show, is really just a clitoris that got exposed early in life to testosterone.

But the penis is so different in size and function from the little nub of the clitoris, you say. Not true! Both have paired bulbs of tissue that swell with sexual stimulation. Both are several inches in size. Wait, what? Did I miss something? Read it again: The clitoris is every bit as large as many a penis; it is simply hidden within the female body and only a very small tip of the organ protrudes externally.

The Bigger Picture

Now that you have familiarized yourself with the various parts, I want to talk about the bigger picture. All of us women need to work on making peace with how our body looks.

Over the last thirty years of clinical practice, so many women have come into my office and nervously giggled as they asked me, "Am I normal down there?" At least 99 percent of the time, their genitals are, in fact, perfectly normal—with the emphasis on perfect! Irregularity and asymmetry are, in fact, totally normal.[13] Variation in color? Normal. Hair in some places you expected and in some you don't want? Normal. Skin that is red, pink, purplish, brown, black, tan, yellow? All normal variations!

Because of the cultural aversion to female genitalia and an awkwardness and squeamishness about discussing anything related to said genitalia, most mothers and fathers never speak to young daughters about their lady parts. Sadly, pediatricians and ob/gyns don't often take the time or feel comfortable broaching the topic. And so perpetuate generations of ignorance and mystery surrounding the female genitalia, as well as sexual inhibitions that contribute to lack of sexual desire and the Bedroom Gap.

The bottom line in the words of the ancient Greek maxim? Know thyself. We all look different—there is no one vulva that is the "right" one—so however you look, you are most likely both totally unique and totally normal down there—I can promise you that.

Making Peace with Your Inhibitions

Most of my patients want something to ignite their desire, some magic libido bullet; when we really dig into what is or isn't happening in the bedroom, it is often just that they are too tired, or that their brains are too full of "other stuff"—and that is what is inhibiting them from being in the moment or really interested in sex.

When it comes to libido, sometimes you are your own worst enemy. Even if you don't have physical reasons for low desire, as we discussed earlier in this chapter, the kinds of inhibitions that take up too much space in our heads because of concerns about body image can lead to huge issues. After all, preventing your own desire from bubbling to the surface might be a bigger issue than not having any desire at all.

Sometimes our inhibitions are not so much about how much energy or focus you have in the moment. Instead, they may relate to body image and body shame, or even to a history of sexual assault or trauma. This can explain why some women don't like foreplay, or don't like parts of their bodies to be touched. Some women want to get under the covers quickly or have sex in the dark. Some women who experienced unwanted arousal during a sexual assault even cringe or are repulsed by sexual arousal itself, as it triggers the shame they felt for becoming aroused during an assault.

The Dual-Control Model

In the late 1990s two researchers at the Kinsey Institute developed the dual-control model of sexual response. This is not just academic mumbo jumbo: It actually describes the mechanism by which your brain and nervous system respond to sexual stimuli (sights, sounds, smells, tastes, sensations, and thoughts). Simply put, they described a series of excitatory and inhibitory pathways in the brain and called them the Sexual Excitation System and the Sexual Inhibition System. These systems are "on call" 24/7, sending signals to the genitals and key parts of the brain to turn on or off, depending on whether it is safe to get turned on, or whether, for example if you could get pregnant or are fooling around with someone you shouldn't, it is better to call off the actions that might lead to trouble.

The reason I want you to know about this is because the inhibitory system can work in our favor to prevent problems. But it can also keep you from getting the sex you want by inhibiting you from getting aroused or orgasming because you are watching your own sexual performance too critically or experiencing performance anxiety or arousal contingency, whereby you can't get aroused unless everything is just right and every sexual stimulus is perfect.

Not only do we need to lose inhibitions to enjoy sex but we also need to be able to focus on our desire and pick up on the sexual cues that lead to arousal. The ability to be in the moment depends on our ability to pay attention to what we're doing. This is true for sex as much as it is for driving, pickle ball, or brain surgery.

How can you increase your own sexual excitement? What turns you on is learned, it is contextual, it is cultural. That is why there is such variation in what turns us on. It doesn't matter what turns women on, or what turns American women on—it only matters what turns *you* on.

Try This

Make a note in your smartphone if you notice you are turned on by something—a smell, a person, a movie scene, a book scene— what is the common thread? Do a little due diligence on yourself this month and jot down some notes. . . . Most importantly, **pay attention!**

How to Increase Your Chances of Enjoyable Sex

As screens compete with face-to-face conversations, and newspapers and books have been crammed into tiny computer screens, and entertainment and information is pressurized into tiny video snippets, we have lost the art of paying attention.

Sexual stimuli, cues, and the nuances of attraction and erotic information require attention. A raised eyebrow, the brush of the back of a hand against a cheek, noticing a muscle here or the faintest smile there. These are the sexy subtleties of flirting, or romance, or tenderness. They lay the foundation of attraction for another person, and they aren't found on twenty-second video reels in your phone— we need to remember to look up from our screens at the person across the couch or table to notice these tiny, glorious moments.

Set the Mood

To have a better chance at getting turned on, you need an appropriate setting. I'm talking about a bedroom free from anger, resentment, and distractions. Clear the air but also clear the room. If clutter, unfolded laundry, work papers, or kids' stuff distract you, remove them from your bedroom. It's okay to prep for sex. Declutter your bedroom so you can declutter your mind. Then add candles, music, room temperature, soft sheets, soft lighting (dimmers are inexpensive to install), a wedge pillow. A little forethought is its own foreplay.

And, speaking of paying attention, no cell phones in the bedroom! This is a death knell to a meaningful sexual encounter. Nothing says "this sex is just so-so" better than picking up your cell phone and scrolling through emails or a social media feed immediately before or after sex.

The next thing you need is sexual stimuli: teasing, laughing, hugging, and touching. Maybe there are some things that mean something to you personally—perhaps you took notes on them in our exercise earlier! The scent of a favorite soap or cologne. A sexy piece of underwear—on you or your partner! Watching a sex scene together. Any kind of foreplay you both enjoy—role-play, toys, oils, foods (do you favor savory or sweet?)—whatever gets you and your partner involved with each other and sets your mind free from the outside world of emails and responsibilities.

Ideally, sexual stimuli in the right setting will pique sexual interests and you'll be open to sex. Once this happens, arousal naturally follows, and this in turn leads to a response to the arousal: desire. The desire for sex then perpetuates the sex play and leads to a satisfying sexual outcome. Remember: It is *normal*, especially in a long-term, multidimensional, and complex relationship, with kids, taxes, work, trash duty, etc., not to be jonesing for sex all the time. But a bit of proactive planning and mindfulness can keep arousal in the picture enough to lead to desire in the moment. And sometimes that's enough.

Try This

Quick tips for a sex jump start:
1. Pinpoint stress source and take action to reduce it
2. Be curious about what pleases you
3. Stop trying to force yourself to want sex
4. Say no to performance anxiety / how sex is "supposed" to be
5. Get to know your body
6. Be affectionate with your partner
7. Stop ruminating about what isn't happening, what it used to be like
8. Focus on intentional touch

Let's Talk About Sex (with Your Partner!)

We have discussed a number of ways to get *yourself* more ready and open to enjoyable sexual experiences, even when you don't feel super in the mood. Now it is time to talk to your partner about how to work on this together.

When I meet with couples, I spend our first couple of sessions mostly listening and having free-form conversations. I want them to offer up their thoughts on what each one thinks is going on. I want to know everything, even if they find it embarrassing to discuss. I want to know about all their issues, whether frustrating, boring, painful, or puerile.

Then I meet individually with the partners so they can share things they might not be comfortable saying in front of each other. I've always marveled at the ease with which people will sometimes unburden themselves of the most intimate details of their lives to a total stranger, including things they can't even say to their sex partner. Couples can have sex together for decades without being able to say a simple thing such as "I don't like that," or "this doesn't feel good," or "that turns me on when you touch me like that."

When I'm alone with a male patient, I learn so much about his needs and wants. Each person is unique, but there are commonalities that bear revealing. Men commonly feel ashamed and attacked outside the bedroom in the course of daily married or partnered life. They tell me that their female spouse is highly critical of everything they do, and that when they elect to do a chore, it is never "done right." I often hear, "Whatever I do, it isn't enough" or "I feel underappreciated."

Moreover, men feel they can't share their fantasies with their partners; they are pretty sure that if they tell them what they see and like from the porn they enjoy, they will be judged critically. So when men don't feel safe, happy, or appreciated, they don't feel they can show vulnerability and ask for what they want. And a complaining partner outside the bedroom is a less desirable partner in bed—this goes for men and women. Men tend to fall back on what they think is "acceptable sex," even if it ends up being pretty dull and unimaginative.

The communication issues don't just fall on the man's side of the equation. Women are complicated too. They want a man to be strong, safe, sturdy, protective. They also want men who are capable of tenderness and communicating their feelings with honesty and vulnerability. But this is hard for any man to pull off gracefully—the two sides seem antithetical.

Furthermore, as we know, women have long been socialized to believe that sex is for a man's pleasure and to satisfy his "needs." They are not taught to ask for what *they* want and often worry that if they were to do so, the behavior would make them seem selfish, promiscuous, even slutty. Nor do they feel comfortable taking on a role in leading, guiding, teaching, or even initiating sex. In other words, "I can't ask for that because I don't know what he'll think about it."

Some women don't know how to ask because they were never given explicit permission to do so. Others feel they shouldn't have to ask. Either way, the outcome is failure in getting women's needs met, and the end result is the perpetuation of unfulfilling sex. This bedroom power structure has existed for millennia and so it has been repeated and reinforced by countless successive generations of heterosexual couples. Even the most powerful, successful women usually abide by this dynamic. Having a clinic in one of the most prestigious university towns in the world, I have been privy to the sexual habits of a very diverse cohort of women. My patients come from every continent and myriad religious and ethnic backgrounds. Many are connected to Princeton University as fellows or visiting professors and are world-renowned in their field. Olympians and Nobel prize winners are overrepresented, but that is exactly what I'm getting at. If any women would feel entitled to smash the gendered sexual roles I'm describing, it would be these titans of academia, sport, art, and finance. They have taken risks and put themselves out there onstage, in sports, in the courtroom, boardroom, classroom, but in the privacy of my office exam room, time and again, they share their sexual frustrations, including the all-too-common "I have to force myself to have sex, for him" mantra. My challenge, in turn, is to change their thinking from "sex in service of male pleasure" to "sex as something also for my pleasure."

What about other sexual couplings? Yes, there are Bedroom Gaps affecting couples outside the heterosexual types. Even with lesbian couples, there are power dynamics. Often, I see one partner, regardless of gender or sexual orientation, assuming a role of caretaker/power player, and the other as the one "taken care of," who feels financially or otherwise obligated to perform sexual servitude even if there is no interest or pleasure in it for her. This power structure can work for some couples but can be problematic when one of the partners gets tired of the roles outside the bedroom and brings this resentment and frustration into it.

Deciding to Have That
First Conversation

One of the first things you can do when you want to improve the state of your sex life is *deciding* to communicate—which is easier said than done. In her book *Smart Sex*, Emily Morse suggests talking about sex regularly (like voting, early and often) to foster a culture of openness and of healthy sex communication: Communication is lubrication, she says.[14] Since most couples pay bills monthly and take out the trash weekly, why not also have a regular check-in about something as important as your sex life? And yet, this very human, very personal and private act, unique in structure and content to every sexual couple, is sometimes never talked about between them.

Before we talk about talking, we need to talk about when, where, and how. Lack of privacy, poor sleep, a recent disagreement, or plain topical awkwardness can be just the impediments you need to never have the talk at all.

Quite possibly the worst time and place to talk about sex? Before or during sex. Nobody wants to feel like they're being critiqued or criticized. Talking about what's working or not will only make your partner defensive or self-conscious. Spectatoring, or watching yourself and your partner's sexual act, destroys your ability to be in the moment. And a talk just before sex would almost definitely invite spectatoring.

There is one exception to this no-sex-talk-when-having-sex rule: the afterglow period. I've talked with couples who love talking about their sex after they finish. They are basking in the flood of dopamine and the rosy, sweaty glow of after sex. They wonder why they don't do this more often. Nothing wrong with that.

But if you're just going through the motions, having sex because your partner wants it or just "getting it over with," you need to find the courage to talk about the sex you are or are not having and about the sex you want. If you are attempting to broach a less-than-glowing review of the sex you're having, consider doing it while taking a walk. Why? Much like a therapists' couch, it is easier for words to come out when you are not also reading a person's facial expressions. On a walk, you are both facing forward. Your partner can hear your words in a more neutral way without the added complication of body language and facial expressions. The body in motion is more relaxed. I find I breathe more deeply because I need to when walking, which promotes further relaxation. Also, any awkward pauses are less awkward if you are multitasking.

Ultimately, whatever works for you is the right answer. If a face-to-face or knee-to-knee conversation gives the talk the focus and gravitas it deserves, then go for it. If a phone call is the only way you can muster the courage to open the sex talk door, then do that. If taking a walk feels easiest, put your walking shoes on. Please just know that I'm a big fan of in-person conversations for important things. And this is an important thing.

How Do You Talk About the Thing No One Likes to Talk About?

So you've figured out when and where. How about I give you some prompts to help you get things started?

- Think about starting on a positive note: "I really enjoyed sex last night, and I would love to hear what I can do to make it great for you as well."
- If you're in a sexual rut, it doesn't hurt to acknowledge that: "It seems sex for us has become a bit challenging. What do you think is the reason for that?"
- Ask open-ended questions: "What do you wish we did more of, sexually speaking?" If your partner demurs because this stuff is awkward, you can restart with something simpler and more specific: "What is it that I do, or don't do but you wish I did, that really turns you on?"
- If you're on a roll and your partner is welcoming the conversation, you can make a specific ask: "I'd like to tell you something I would like more of in our sex life," or "Something I wish you did more often/we could try together is . . ."
- Discuss trying new things: "Would you consider X?" where X might be the use of a toy, lube, a different position, a throuple, or an erotic couples massage.
- If the conversation is really open, you can get into some more difficult stuff too, the kinds of questions or concerns we really try to avoid, like pain during sex, bleeding during sex, odor, lack of orgasm, or ongoing avoidance of sex. This could even be a real truthful conversation about how to approach having sex after surgery or sex after an affair.

- If you just can't muster the courage or find the words or the sex-positive tone, try listening to a podcast with sexual content alone or with your partner to get comfortable with terms, phrases, and hearing about the topic *together*.
- This is super important, and the more vulnerable and curious and open you are to conversation about sex, and the more conversations you have with your partner, the better your sex will become.

What If I'm Not Ready to Talk Specifics or Play Out Sexual Fantasies?

Maybe you're not ready to talk about sex. Or perhaps you aren't really ready to have sex at all. The first thing you need to do is figure out whether your roadblock is relational or situational. If your relationship is struggling, talking with a third person or even taking a course such as a condensed communication workshop like Imago Relationship Therapy can help kick-start honest conversations about what's going on between you.[15]

Sometimes these kinds of conversations are opportunities just to say *one* difficult thing to each other out loud: "I really hate sex at night because I am tired," or "I have never really liked it when you lick my ear. It annoys me and doesn't turn me on." But it could also be deeper issues such as "your mother living with us is making me resentful." Your relationship challenges might be playing out in the bedroom, but before you can fix the sex, you might need to get to the root cause of what's been hurting your relationship health.

If the issue is in part or whole a situational one, the problem-solving will look a little different. No privacy? Find a time in the week when you might be able to have sex without teens or toddlers or your mother-in-law around. Or if you can pull it off, treat yourself to a getaway for just one night. It doesn't have to be far flung or expensive. An AirBnB or local inn where you can focus on being together rather than sightseeing may be more conducive to rekindling intimacy than somewhere exotic.

Stress from your job, family, or financial issues? These are tricky to just make disappear, but remember—regular sex lowers blood pressure and reduces stress. It can also strengthen the feeling that you and your partner are in this together, and that you have his/her love and support to get you through a stressful time. So more sex—even if it feels like the last thing you can manage to make time for—might actually benefit you during stressful periods.

Faking It Until You Make It

I would never advocate faking pleasure—the tried and true and, to be honest, worn-out expectation that women fake orgasms has helped to get us into this mess of a Bedroom Gap in the first place, after all! But I don't think faking desire is the worst idea. What I mean by that is that there are some easy ways to get yourself into a position of feeling a little more sexual desire. Treating the source of your sexual pain, getting to know yourself, your body, and your turn-ons—and those of your partner's—while also turning your To-Do list off and your Do It list on—all these things can spark desire and lead to a little more interest in fitting sex in your life.

Give yourself a little grace. No one expects *every* night to be a tear your clothes off and have sex on the kitchen floor kind of night. If you are willing to be open—to setting a mood, to communicating openly, even regularly, with your partner, to finding the time to be with each other—the sexual payoffs will come (pun, absolutely).

Once you have kick-started a bit more sexual desire for your-self, the next hill to conquer is to rewrite your own sexual script, to reshape the sex you are having with your increased sexual pleasure as the intended outcome. To close the Bedroom Gap, we have to under-stand its components: gaps between partners in desire, in pleasure, in orgasm. We've done a deep dive into desire, now let's look at both pleasure and orgasm.

Chapter 5

Pleasure

Modern society has a problem with, almost an aversion to, pleasure. And I am not sure we are even aware of it. Pleasure can be a feeling, a source of delight, an activity for relaxation or enjoyment. We talk a big game about Me Time and Down Time, but we first world folk are not optimizing our lives for pleasure. As sex therapist and podcaster Emily Morse says in her book *Smart Sex*, we tend to "optimize for growth instead—productivity growth, financial growth, social media growth, professional growth."[1]

We are so tethered to our phones, our schedules, video meetings, calendars, endless errands, the daily grind, commutes, and committee meetings. We feel good when we get through our to-do list, when we get stuff done. We praise the frenzied parents who can manage a double income household while working eighty-hour work weeks. We don't really tip our hats to those folks who make time to smell the roses, take a pay cut, and skip the race to the brass ring. What if we made pleasure a priority, a goal, an achievement unto itself?

Guilty Pleasures

I'd like you to reframe how you see and value pleasure and to consider a reprioritization of it in your life. Not just sexual pleasure, but pleasure as a concept.

My mom turned eighty this year and still struggles with the guilt of her own pleasure. She was, for seventy-four of her eighty years, a card-carrying member of the camp of women who think enjoyment is for someone else, that pleasure is a selfish, shameful concept. She used to sigh-complain-boast that she never got around to drinking her morning tea until the afternoon and had not had a full meal sitting down in years. "I have too much to do, too many people need me," she would say. Then, six years ago, she was diagnosed with multiple myeloma, a rare cancer in the blood marrow.

Soon after her diagnosis, my mom had an epiphany. She was racing around to nowhere, striving for some domestic martyrdom, but for what? For nothing. She realized that it was okay to do things that brought her joy, even if her to-do list went unfinished or my dad ate—cue the dead Greek relatives turning over in their graves— canned soup. While it is unfortunate that it took a cancer diagnosis to shake her fundamental belief that as a female, a wife, and a mother, she did not deserve to think about herself first, it has been amazing to watch her personal growth and the realization that pleasure is indeed hers to claim.

These days my mother giggles more, takes online courses about things she's "always wanted to learn," flirts with my ninety-year-old dad, shares off-color jokes, and eats the cookie dough she always told us not to eat ("there's raw eggs in that!"). She reminds us that Sting is "still hot!" and that she thinks professional soccer players have "beautiful bodies." She has a whimsy, even a devilish prankster streak that she kept buried for decades under piles of laundry, mountains of productivity (she was a successful real estate developer and owned an antiques business), heaps of putting others first, shitloads of societal pressure to have a perfectly spotless house. Her home is still clean and neat, but now she gives herself room for pleasure.

That air-brushed Martha Stewart photo shoot life some women strive for is antithetical to the spontaneous joy of pleasure-generating activities, including sexual pleasure. Sex is sweaty, messy, guttural, and real. And apart from truly asexual humans, we *all* do it.[2] Spontaneous sex sometimes butts up against deadlines and appointments and life order. It is the Id to the Superego of Martha's one thousand thread count, nonstick, tufted, trompe l'oeil life that many women feel is the apex of femalehood.

So, ladies, learn it now, or rather unlearn it, now. Imperfection—whether a missed promotion or burned shakshuka—is real, it is inescapable, it is totally fine. And pleasure is yours to claim. Once you really believe it and can practice it, then sexual pleasure is more possible.

Try This

Naming **your guilt-free** (not guilty) **pleasure**. What brings you pleasure? What makes you smile, laugh, or just relax a bit? What would you name as your "guilty pleasure?" Mine is getting outside in nature, appreciating a new bloom in my garden or a squirrel industriously shuttling acorns. I also love the creativity of cooking a meal for fun (as opposed to the 1,092 or so standard meals a year that are not my version of fun)—the herbs, spices, scents, the anticipation of tasting a new recipe or the satisfied sigh of tasting an old staple well crafted. What's yours?

Why is it so hard for women to embrace pleasure as healthy and nutritious, as opposed to guilty, even shameful, especially when it comes to sex? Why do we call taking an hour for ourselves to take a walk or eat a food that we love or watch an episode of something we enjoy a *"guilty* pleasure?" I don't know, but I assume it is all part of the female nurturer caregiver selfless martyr puritanical work ethic bullshit we have all been fed. Let's exchange "guilty" for "guilt-free" pleasure. Pleasure is healthy. Please say that three times. Out loud. *Pleasure is healthy. Pleasure is healthy. Pleasure is healthy.* Put a sticky note on your bathroom mirror that says: Pleasure is healthy.

Pleasure Hierarchies

Modern society has implicit rules about who gets to be first in line to receive pleasure. If you ask pretty much any woman, this is obvious. Why is it that so many women feel they have to ask, even nag their male partner to do household tasks?[3] "Honey, can you put down the remote and give me a hand scrubbing the pots?" said pretty much no *man*, ever. The prioritization of male pleasure is relentlessly, but insidiously, fed to us in the media, through generational modeling and in the very way we learn about gendered sex roles. Sex—for men—is a conquest, an entitlement, a biological need. For women, it's an obligation, or a gift to a partner, or something to barter for money or popularity, heck, for a night off from the kids. Any wonder why it also, too often, ends up being a chore? The feminist philosopher Kate Manne examines the gendered hierarchy of entitlement in her must-read book *Entitled: How Male Privilege Hurts Women.* She explores why men believe they are entitled to, among other things, sex from women, and why they often struggle to intuit that women have needs as well, including the need to consent to sex, to desire sex, and to get pleasure from sex.[4]

What Gets in the Way of Pleasure?

What you bring to the bedroom in terms of how you relate to being a sexual person is a mix of past and present, a psychological formulation of sexual values learned in childhood largely from parents but overlaid with sexual ideas learned at school, from friends, in media, in sex ed class, and from your uncle's *Penthouse* magazine.

Then, as you become a sexual being yourself, your ideas and your own sexual scripting is further shaped by your early sexual encounters and refined by subsequent ones. Each of your sex partners taught you something about sex. In some cases you learned together, in others your partner taught you or vice versa. Sometimes, the learning was by negative example. We come to a sexual relationship with baggage and background from our past, blended with who we are and how we are in the here and now. This complicated combination of past and present factors will affect what happens in your bedroom tonight, and every night.

What are the sexual stumbling blocks that get in the way of pleasure and make us averse to sex, or hesitant to share our wants even with a long-term partner? What factors make us slide quickly under the covers, reflexively turn on the TV, or turn off the light and turn away, or cause us to limit ourselves sexually to certain behaviors, acts, positions?

Emily Morse describes three emotional factors likely to "undermine your erotic potential" as the Pleasure Thieves: stress, trauma, and shame.[5]

Stress
We've discussed how stress hinders desire and distracts us from getting in the mood for sex. But stress also has a profound effect on our ability to feel pleasure.

Stress can be acute or chronic. The acute version can make it difficult to be in the moment because our mind is focused on the acute stressor, say a costly fender bender earlier that day. Chronic stress, such as caring for an aging parent or a partner with severe depression, kills our sexual buzz in perhaps more profound ways. Chronic stress means prolonged increased production of cortisol, which is a burden on the adrenal glands and is associated with anxiety and depression.

Stress, whether acute or chronic, activates the sympathetic nervous system. You know that stomach lurching, or chest tightening, or sweaty palm feeling? You can't really feel sexual pleasure when the sympathetic nervous system is engaged.

The parasympathetic system, on the other hand, says, "Relax. Enjoy. Take your time." It is antithetical to the sympathetic system. It is the parasympathetic system that allows us to feel pleasure. Stress = Sympathetic. Pleasure = Parasympathetic.

While there is no easy way to switch off or switch between these two competing systems, we do have ways to tamp down the sympathetic type and reduce how stress affects us, making room for parasympathetic activation. And we don't need expensive medications or therapy. Three simple things you already have in your arsenal can reduce stress to allow for pleasure in life (and in sex!): exercise, breathing, and social interaction.

Exercise: I am not saying you need to embark on triathlete level training, but movement of almost any kind will improve your energy level, your life outlook, your lifespan, and yes, your enjoyment of sex.

Breathing: Breathing exercises are simple and effective stress reduction techniques. Deep breathing stimulates the vagus nerve, which is a major player in the parasympathetic system. So deep breathing literally is a way to turn on your parasympathetic nervous system. Aaaahhhh.

Social interaction: Socializing can reduce stress in many ways. Whether your version is hanging out with friends, mentoring a coworker, volunteering at a homeless shelter, bringing a cake to your church group or wine to your book group, engaging with other humans in loving and generous ways is good for us. Positive social interactions release endorphins, are an antidote to loneliness, boost self-esteem, and can give life a sense of purpose and belonging, making room for pleasure to flourish.

Let's Breathe!

Easy breathing exercises that do not require a Yogi, a Himalayan singing bowl, or incense can really reset your frame of mind. For any of these, sit up straight, pull your torso up from your pelvis, relax your shoulders down away from your ears, and focus only on the movement of the air into your lungs and out of your body.

1. **4-4-4 breathing:** Breathe in through your mouth for 4 seconds, hold for 4 seconds, breathe out through your nose for 4 seconds. Easy.

2. **4-7-8 breathing:** Again, breathe in for 4 seconds but hold for 7 seconds (or even 9 if you can do it). Then take a long, prolonged exhale for 8 seconds to really push all the air out of the lungs.

3. **Focused breathing:** Breathe in and out as above, or just equally inhale and exhale, but focus on imagery or a word. Alternatively, lie down and put one hand on your belly to feel the belly button rise and fall. Focus on the up-and-down movement of the diaphragm.

Trauma

Trauma is the most insidious of the pleasure thieves. Too many of us have experienced a traumatic event that interferes with our willingness to be vulnerable sexually. For some, it was inadvertently seeing a sexual act or being touched inappropriately at a young age and having negative feelings associated with the event. For others, it is a negative, nonconsensual, or forced initial sexual encounter. A 2019 article in the *Journal of the American Medical Association* reported that about one in sixteen women, or 6.5 percent of women, reported their initial sexual encounter as forced, and the mean age of this encounter was 15.6 years. Disturbingly, over 40 percent reported being physically restrained, but even more reported verbal or psychological pressure.[6]

We know that trauma greatly impacts our ability to be vulnerable, sexually open, curious, and fun loving, which can hamstring a sex life and create or worsen a Bedroom Gap at any age. Therapy, and there are therapists specifically trained to deal with trauma, is a critical component of getting yourself unstuck from the hindrances of childhood or adult trauma.

Shame

Shame is a real sexual buzzkill. It is one of those useless, unhelpful emotions that we know we don't need but can't easily shed. Sexual shame plays out in bedrooms as sexual dysfunction, whether as an inability or reduced ability to orgasm, erectile difficulties, or feelings of unattractiveness.

A common cause of sexual shame for women is vaginal odor. One patient, Susan, told me, "Every time, with every partner, the fear that my odor is going to be a turn off consumes me. It's all I can think about whenever someone starts to move down my body. And once someone starts touching my underwear, forget it. All I want to do is squirm away. Or apologize for the smell. Or take a shower, again." Some odor is normal. If you feel your odor is very strong ask a clinician to evaluate. Strong, unpleasant odor is often due to bacterial vaginosis and is easy to treat.

Another common source of shame is a woman's fear of what her anatomy looks like, that her partner will find an ingrown hair unattractive, or the wiggling dangling larger labia on one side odd-looking. Be comfortable in your body, imperfections and all, and don't let shame creep into your bedroom, robbing you of the joy you deserve.

The third example of shame I hear from my patients is that of rejecting sexual requests from a partner, most commonly anal and sometimes oral sex. Do what you want, not what your partner wants. It is healthy to have an open mind and to try new things, but performing sex acts you really don't want to doesn't serve you or deepen the relationship.

How Do You Overcome Sexual Shame?

1. Find a behavioral health professional specifically trained to talk about sex. AASECT, the American Association of Sexuality Educators, Counselors, and Therapists is the best place to look.[7]
2. Get educated! It is never too late to learn more about sex, trauma, anatomy, relationships, communication skills. Education helps shed the shame, wherever it came from.
3. Behavioral therapies such as cognitive reappraisal allow you to reframe your feelings about sex so you can flip the negative thoughts to positive ones.

Spectatoring

One additional pleasure thief I would add is spectatoring, basically self-observation during sex, which can cause Bedroom Gaps in a relationship by limiting one's ability to fully be "in the moment." If you are busy judging the sex, worrying about how you look or sound or smell, you rob yourself of the ability to love the experience.

How Your First Time
Affects Pleasure Downstream

There has been much hullabaloo over the concept of "losing [one's] virginity." I say the focus should not be on whether you are a virgin (remember we are talking about a flimsy bit of hymenal tissue) but under what circumstances said virginity was lost. The nature of one's first sexual encounter, especially for women, shapes their attitudes toward sex for decades to come. In an excellent article in *Forbes*, psychologist Mark Travers describes the long-term effects of our first sexual encounter on our well-being and future sexual identity.[8] Travers shares how having *agency* over that first sexual experience is an important predictor of future sexual health. A *negative* first sexual encounter is associated with feelings of shame (there it is again!) and guilt (driven by cultural dogma) and results in higher rates of sexual difficulties later in life.

A *positive* first sexual experience, for those who are lucky enough to have had one, can launch us properly in our sexual lives, feeling more confident and comfortable about sex, and perhaps enabling us to understand that sex is a lifetime learning project, not something we need to somehow master from the start. (Remember this point when we discuss how the Dutch teach sex ed.) Alas, the gendered Bedroom Gap starts early. Research shows that more men report positive first sexual experiences than women, perhaps because the orgasm rate for men is higher than for women in their first sexual experiences, or because women may be pressured into their first experience or experience pain.

The Neurochemistry of Pleasure

Now that we know some of the obstacles, let's talk about how brain chemistry can work with or against our sexual pleasure.

When people talk about chemistry between two people, there really is something to that. We are products of our own neurochemistry. Our behaviors and passions and some of the biggest decisions, mistakes, and moments of our lives occur because of minute actions of neurochemicals in the tiniest little nerve cells in our brains.

The brain is the stage upon which the chemical and hormonal actors practice their craft. Let's look at what is happening between the ears—at a brain chemistry level—to better explain what happens between the covers. The chemical actors in our own passion play include:

Dopamine: The Exciter

Dopamine (DA) is dope—it is what makes us seek out pleasure. Dopamine gets released when we enjoy something, or even when we are merely anticipating the enjoyment or seeking it out, say, looking for someone to meet at a bar or club or walking to our favorite gelateria.

Things that positively affect DA release include testosterone, sexual stimuli such as the shower head aimed at our vulva, the brush of someone's hand against our skin, thighs touching at a movie theater date, orgasm (duh), even music. Things that hinder the release of DA include stress (increased cortisol opposes dopamine release), anemia, or low magnesium levels. Dopamine also thrives on novelty and is released more frequently when something is new. Novelty-related dopamine release is what makes us chronically curious, or needing to scroll, or buy new things, or have new sex partners. Some lovers are serial monogamists, wanting one partner at a time but always wanting a new partner; others become bored from sex with one partner and seek out multiple partners simultaneously, looking for their next sexual dopamine fix. It is also why the dopamine boost of trying something new or switching up your sex routine can give you and your partner a great feeling.

It turns out that dopamine gets released not only when we are in love but also when we get dumped and are longing for that lost love. The biological anthropologist Helen Fisher spent her career studying the biology of love, including its neurochemistry.[9] In 2006 she found that cells in the ventral tegmental area (VTA) of the brain are involved in love-related dopamine release.[10] MRI images showed that these VTA cells are at play not only when we are "in love" but also when love is rejected. They also can be responsible for the sometimes obsessive actions of rejected lovers, and they are also involved with orgasm, motivation, reward, cognition, and other behaviors. Dopamine has even been shown to play a role in our initial attraction to someone, to forming long-term attachment to a partner, and in who we prefer as a mate.[11] Crazy stuff!

Serotonin: The Satisfier

Serotonin is the neurochemical flip side to dopamine. It is associated with relaxation, a feeling of contentment, a life cup that is seen as half full rather than half empty. It is the herbal tea to dopamine's double espresso. It's how you want your brain to feel when heading to sleep, but not necessarily when trying to get your mojo up for sex.

Too much serotonin can lower sex drive, which is why men and women who take selective serotonin reuptake inhibitors (SSRIs)—

for depression, anxiety, OCD, and even to reduce menopausal symptoms—often lose interest in sex. The SSRIs keep the mood faucet in your brain dripping a steady stream of serotonin. While this helps you feel better, it also makes it harder for dopamine to do its job. You might have fewer hot flashes, or your panic attacks are less frequent, but you also could care less whether you have sex with your new Tinder date or your husband.

If you have SSRI-associated low libido, consider switching to SNRIs, which increase norepinephrine instead of serotonin and may reduce libido less than the SSRIs. Or try one of the antidepressants below, which also have fewer negative effects on libido:[12]

- Bupropion
- Mirtazapine
- Vilazodone
- Vortioxetine
- Nefazodone[13]
- Amitriptyline

Oxytocin: The Cuddler

Oxytocin is yet another neurochemical at play in your sex life. Oxytocin gets released after orgasm and when you are lactating; it promotes feelings of bonding and intimacy. Cuddling is a big oxytocin-mediated activity. Oxytocin is also released with nipple stimulation, which may explain why some women really love attention paid to their nipples during sex.

Prolactin: The Relaxer

Prolactin is responsible for milk production in lactating females, but we also release prolactin during orgasm. Our prolactin levels stay elevated for about an hour after coitus.[14] Prolactin can impact the refractory period—the time from having an orgasm to being able to have another one. It also makes us sleepy, which is why some of us feel really sleepy after climaxing. An interesting fact: Prolactin release after orgasm with a sex partner is 400 percent greater than prolactin released after orgasm from masturbation.[15]

Why have I bothered telling you about all these tiny chemicals in the brain? Because they affect our behavior, whether it is sex drive or falling in or out of love. These neurochemicals—dopamine, serotonin, oxytocin, and prolactin—also work in parallel with the sex steroids—estrogen, progesterone, testosterone—that we know affect sexual desire.

Now let's zero in on the cherry atop the ice cream sundae of sex: the orgasm. Let's explore why orgasms occur differently for men and women, why we fake orgasms, how to have an orgasm, and how to reframe sex without orgasm.

Chapter 6

The Orgasm Gap

The orgasm gap—the marked difference in frequency of orgasms between men and women in heterosexual sexual encounters—is a subset of the Bedroom Gap. Both gaps perfectly exemplify what gender inequality looks like from a sexual perspective.

So much of who we are sexually is dictated by sexual scripts we learn from peers, prior generations, the media (especially porn), and even parents. Do women have fewer orgasms because of anatomy, or a partner's competency, or is it all in our head?

Mind the Gaps

There are five types of orgasm gaps to consider as a framework for understanding the orgasm gap:

1. Between men and women
2. Between women engaged in partnered sex versus masturbation

3. Between women engaged in sex with other women versus with men. Here we can learn from sexual outcomes in bisexual women, since they have partnered sex with both men and women. In one study looking at the propensity to orgasm in bisexual women, orgasm was nine times more likely with the sex partner being female than male.[1]

4. Between women engaged in casual sex versus relationship sex. The orgasm gap is wider in casual sex as opposed to committed relationship sex. One study found that the orgasm rate for women in a committed relationship was 68 percent but only 10 percent with hookup sex. And in fact, first-time hookup sex is about 50 percent less likely to result in orgasm for either gender than relationship sex.[2]

5. An age-related orgasm gap. Orgasm for both sexes wanes with age, likely related to reduced rates of sexual fantasy and desire for sex, as well as vascular and nerve-ending changes that come with age.

Now let's look at two major influences on orgasm for both sexes, intercourse (PIV sex) and porn.

PIV Sex and Orgasm

As a culture, we overvalue penis-in-vagina (PIV) sex as the pinnacle of sex. This concept is so accepted that women don't question its central role in the sexual act, even if it negatively impacts their pleasure and orgasm. That sex equals penile penetration is reinforced by our own linguistic choices: The words "sex" and "intercourse" are pretty much interchangeable. When former President Bill Clinton emphatically announced to the American public that he "did not have sex with that woman!," referring to his sexual encounters with Monica Lewinsky, he knew that he could claim some degree of innocence because there had been no PIV sex. There had been lots of other sexy stuff—including using a cigar as a proxy for the presidential penis—but since no intercourse had occurred, he was claiming there had been no "sex."

PIV sex tends to be disproportionately satisfying to the person who owns the P. In fact, women can orgasm more quickly and more predictably when they are alone. When flying solo, women report having an orgasm 95 percent of the time. But when a male partner is involved, the chance of an orgasm drops to around 65 percent. Women on average need just four minutes to climax if we remove the male partner from the experience; once there is penis pleasing to worry about, female orgasms take on average thirteen to twenty-one minutes to materialize. The likelihood of a female orgasm seems inversely proportional to having a penis in the room. The negligible orgasm gap in the lesbian community is proof that the dearth of female orgasms during a male partnered sexual experience is not due to faulty clitoral wiring. No, the LGBTQ+ lack of orgasm gap tells us that it is gender roles and sexual expectations—*not* anatomy or capacity for pleasure—that governs and guides who orgasms in heterosexual sex.

How Often an Orgasm Occurs During a Sexual Experience[3]

Heterosexual men 95%
Homosexual men 89%
Bisexual men 88%
Homosexual women 86%
Bisexual women 66%
Heterosexual women 65%

As long as PIV sex remains a heterosexual imperative, the orgasm gap will persist across generations and continents, despite feminist declarations of new progressive attitudes and demands for sexual equality.

The Porn Effect

Is porn friend or foe? My views swing and sway, from a longtime loathing of pornography as the source of all evil and the degrading, for-profit use of women for male sexual pleasure to a begrudging acceptance of it as an inescapable part of human experience. I have even come to (wince) appreciate the role of porn in broadening the sexual education of men and women. The pornographic depiction (through a mostly male-directed lens) of a "typical" female sexual experience, which tends to be whittled down to dramatic moaning and writhing, then orgasming within ten seconds of penile penetration, has caused widespread misinformation among men and women. Because of porn, many men and women believe this is how sex should be, how sex should look, how women should sound, how (quickly and consistently) female orgasms happen; they also believe that aggressive, repetitive penile thrusting is the key to unlocking a woman's orgasmic potential. Wrong. Wrong. All wrong, as you already know from Chapter 2 and, well, probably from your own life.

Porn, with its reductive, insulting, and blatantly misogynistic titles, corny music, money shots, and abundance of facials, is the billboard messenger for male sexual fantasy writ very very large.[4] It is a megaphone shout out of the whispered messages we have been fed about who we should be, sexually. And it is a major contributor to failed expectations, relational discontent, and Bedroom Gaps everywhere.

But porn is only the most flagrant example of Bedroom Gap–yielding sexual scripts, putting the "finishing touches"—blow jobs and anal and facials—"on a narrative of sex and relationships that most of us received well before our first porn experience."[5] Take any contemporary rom-com. The sex messages are abundant and predictable: (1) Male-initiated romance is the norm; (2) Masturbation is taboo for women but okay for men; (3) The best lovers intuitively know all the right moves with no discussion; (4) Nice/desirable girls have had few partners and don't sleep around, but they just "know" how to have great sex; and (5) Women climax from PIV sex. These messages are all reinforced and repeated ad nauseum, and we have watched and internalized them since we were kids. Some of them are contradictory and mutually exclusive, by the way: Is sex taboo or glorified? Shameful or powerful? Answer: Both.

If we look at porn with a statistics mindset, we can glean a lot of what we need to know simply by looking at the orgasm frequency of the male and female actors we spend an alarming number of hours watching. Researchers report that in pornographic videos, 76–78 percent of men reach orgasm (I would have guessed 100 percent) while only 17–18 percent of women do so onscreen; significantly, these female orgasms largely result from penile or anal penetrative sex.[6] In fact, looking at PornHub's fifty-most viewed videos of all time, we find that in the videos where women are shown reaching orgasm, only 25 percent involve some form of direct or indirect clitoral stimulation.[7]

If men are taught how to have sex mainly from porn and in the media, women are getting their acting cues from the same (wildly inaccurate) sources. The result is widespread faking of orgasm and sexual pleasure in general. Unfortunately, women faking orgasms perpetuates the miseducation for men that women should be able to climax from vaginal penetration.

So don't blame the men: They are taking cues from the media, from porn, and from their partners! If a woman moans and screams when she is not really having an orgasm, studies show most men will overestimate the number of orgasms their female partners have—and this gives men the wrong idea that they're doing it right. Men also consistently underestimate how often women are faking it.[8] All these issues just increase the orgasm gap, and other gaps too—in communication, in understanding, in pleasure.

Unfortunately, some of the messages porn perpetuates are dangerous. The proliferation of porn into every corner of society is at least in part to blame for the recent sexual trend in choking—porn has normalized choking as au courant sex play.[9] Men want to try it and women feel like they're supposed to enjoy it. But strangulation tends to be very uneven from a gender standpoint (most often, it is the woman being strangled), and it is potentially dangerous behavior that has led to deaths from asphyxiation.

Even if the behavior porn encourages isn't on the super-risky end of the spectrum, it is still dangerous in and of itself. Watching excessive amounts of porn can have negative effects on a relationship, fostering a loss of trust and lack of emotional closeness with a partner. Porn addiction can lead to an unrealistic understanding about sex. Sex then becomes performative (spectatoring!), and the partners of a sex addict can never live up to the standards of pornographic depictions of sex. Watching porn excessively can be a setup for loneliness, social isolation, and sexual dysfunction. Much like a drug addict needs more and more of a drug to get high, a porn addict develops a desensitization of the brain's reward system. This makes it harder to feel pleasure or achieve erection or orgasm in real-life sexual encounters. Is your partner watching a lot of porn or a known porn addict? If so, this is next-level Bedroom Gap, and you need to get him/her support, such as provided by one of the many twelve-step treatment programs and of course get support for yourself as well. You can't close a Bedroom Gap like this alone.

Self-Love

Closing the orgasm gap starts with looking at self-love. Women who masturbate (starting at any age) are more knowledgeable about their body and know how to elicit pleasure, including pleasure from orgasm. Whether they are straight or gay, single or partnered, masturbation helps women feel comfortable experiencing physical pleasure, letting go of stress, shame, and intrusive thoughts, and yes, getting to orgasm.

What if you've never masturbated? Is it too late? Never. It is never too late to get to know your body and to close your orgasm gap. (If you're ready to start right this second, skip ahead to the next chapter for a primer on masturbation!)

Orgasm Variations

The variations in orgasm from woman to woman and from one partner and position to the next are extremely frustrating. Confused couples come to my office with questions such as "What's the problem? Why me? Why with him/her? Why now?" Some women never have an orgasm. Ever. Some have orgasms only in certain positions, or only with certain partners. Some women have multiple orgasms and even these orgasms vary from several in rapid succession, which are genitally focused, to a few deep full body orgasms. Orgasms occur most predictably from stimulation of the external glans of the clitoris but can also occur from stimulation of the G-spot along the top wall of the vagina, the A-spot (also along the anterior vaginal wall but deeper inside), the cervix, or even non-genital areas such as the nipples. Women are full of potential areas to stimulate and ways to achieve orgasm.

Do you know that females can ejaculate? Female ejaculate resulting from an orgasm is about two ounces of fluid, similar to male ejaculate but minus the sperm. Some women "squirt" and others don't.

"Squirting" refers to the release of fluid from the urethra during orgasm; this fluid is a mixture of urine and fluid from the Skene's glands—remember those paired, "Beautiful and Sexy" glands flanking the urethral opening from Chapter 1?

Achieving Orgasm in PIV Sex

Wish you could improve pleasure for yourself during penetrative sex? Four specific techniques women use to enhance pleasure during PIV sex described by one study include angling (87.5 percent of respondents), rocking (76 percent), shallowing (84 percent), and pairing (69.7 percent). The nitty gritty of each:

- **Angling:** Rotating, raising, or lowering the pelvis/hips during penetration to adjust where inside the vagina the toy or penis rubs and what it feels like.
- **Rocking:** If the penis or sex toy is kept inside the vagina rather than moved in and out, there is constant clitoral stimulation from the base of the penis or toy.
- **Shallowing:** Penetrative touch just inside the entrance of the vagina—not on the outside, but also not deep inside—with a fingertip, sex toy, penis tip, tongue, or lips. Remember the labia minora and the vestibule are loaded with nerve endings and are part of the sensory experience of sexual arousal.
- **Pairing:** When a woman herself (solo pairing) or her partner (partner pairing) reaches down to stimulate her clitoris with a finger or sex toy at the same time as her vagina is being penetrated.[10]

Faking It

Blame porn. Blame media. Blame society. Regardless of the reason, we know that women's expectations of sex rarely line up with reality, which leads us to be dishonest, with others and with ourselves, about what we like, what we don't like, and what we want. In other words, we lie about sex. We do. We alter the sexual version of ourselves to fit some idealized vision of what we think a partner wants: sexy but not slutty, chaste but not frigid. Or some blended version, depending on what we *think* our partner is looking for. We also tend not to ask for what we want in bed, out of politeness, embarrassment, or even just lack of knowledge about what we enjoy. And we fake orgasms. Pretty often, it turns out.

Why do women "fake it"?

- Orgasm is part of our expected sexual script.
- We want to show a partner that we are enjoying sex.
- We choose to have some control over the situation.
- We want to bring a sexual encounter to a conclusion . . .
  - because the sex is subpar or
  - because we have been pressured or forced to have a sexual experience we weren't interested in.
- To bridge a Bedroom Gap between expectation (from culture, media, myth) and reality.

One common reason for faking an orgasm is because *talking about sex is difficult*. The three most common reasons for not talking with a partner about sex include not wanting to hurt a partner's feelings (42.4 percent), not feeling comfortable going into detail (40.2 percent), and embarrassment (37.7 percent).[11]

Men can fake orgasms as well, and quite convincingly. While an average of 58 percent of women have faked orgasm, 25 percent of men admit to having done so, by pretending to ejaculate onto a sheet, into their hand, into their partner's body, or into a condom.[12] These statistics, in my opinion, are akin to wild guesses. They could be slightly off or vastly underreporting the real picture. Orgasm faking occurs between female partners as well. Sex therapist Christine Claypoole notes that with lesbian couples, a power dynamic can exist (whether personality driven or economically based) that leads to sexual behaviors that include faking orgasms, often for the same reasons gay men and heterosexual couples fake orgasms.[13]

Pop Quiz

When a woman fakes orgasm, is she:

    A. Letting herself down
    B. Betraying the feminist movement
    C. Preserving male ego
    D. Claiming control over a situation (getting through meh sex)
    E. All of the above

Orgasms, Testosterone, and Your Health
One reason to opt for real as opposed to fake orgasms is that orgasms offer numerous health benefits, including:

- Stress and anxiety reduction
- Better sleep
- Increased relaxation
- The growth of neurons in the hippocampus
- Decreased pain, including menstrual pain
- A boosted immune system, through the release of natural killer cells and leukocytes

According to urologist and podcaster Kelly Casperson, orgasms can also help pass kidney stones![14] Regular orgasms have even been linked to longevity.[15] So, we want to do everything we can to encourage having more of them—real, not fake ones! One solution that we aren't taking advantage of yet, medically speaking, is using topical testosterone applied to the clitoris to facilitate and intensify your orgasm. Applied regularly (not prior to sex) to the clitoris, testosterone restores and maintains blood vessels and nerve endings, which are needed for sexual function.[16] The clitoris is the only part of the body whose sole function is pleasure, so why not maintain its health just as you would maintain your overall health? Clitoral health is a part of sexual health, after all, and the care and management of both should be a lifelong endeavor. I tell my patients that topical testosterone for the clitoris (used sparingly) and topical vaginal estrogen should be used by anyone with said anatomy and, like seat belts and sunblock, can be safely used forever.[17]

The Meh-gasm
On the flip side, we need to be a little less orgasm obsessed. What if our orgasms are mediocre, wimpy, not worth the effort? Author Lux Alptraum shares in her book *Faking It*, "Women get taught that orgasm is a mandatory requirement for good sex and that it's also supposed to be mind-blowingly fantastic. . . . If you're not readily orgasmic, or if your definition of good sex doesn't necessarily involve your own orgasmic release, or your orgasms aren't as earth shattering as they're 'supposed' to be, [women mistakenly believe] the problem is with you and not with the cultural narrative itself." She also writes, "Our intense romanticization of the grand climax isn't just inaccurate but actively works to prevent people . . . from enjoying sex."[18] There is such an intense focus on an incredible orgasm as the purpose

and end goal of sex that anything less feels like a failure to a woman and her partner. Admitting your orgasms happen but are mediocre is either an insult to your partner's sexual skill level (got to protect that delicate male ego!) or akin to admitting you aren't "good at sex." None of us wants to willingly embrace that! So, the so-so orgasm stays undiscussed.

The underwhelming orgasm is more common than Hollywood, porn, or really everything we (think we) know about sex seems to suggest. What's a girl to do? If you are harboring a good amount of negativity around your present sex life, including a so-so orgasm capacity, I invite you to consider a shift in perspective to sex sans orgasm. What? Why? Because even if your version of sex does not include ending with a mind-blowing orgasm, if *you* feel fulfilled, then you are living your best sexual life. A lack of orgasm is only a problem if you deem it so.

This is not to say that you should continue having middling sex, without asking for what you want. If a toe-curling orgasm is what you want, then work toward that. But if you are enjoying sex with your partner—even if you aren't having an earth-shattering orgasm to close the encounter out—and you are feeling fulfilled and satisfied, then stop worrying about how anyone else thinks sex should look for you. Anyone who has taken a wine tasting course knows the best wine is the one you like, not the one that *Wine Spectator* rates the highest.

Sex Without Orgasm? Really?

What's so great about non–orgasm focused sex? For many of my patients, once they unhook themselves from the notion that they *have to* have an orgasm, they feel liberated, free to enjoy sex for its own sake rather than as a means to an end. My patient Kerry and I had a great discussion about this recently. She rattled off some really spot-on reasons why she loves taking the Big O out of her sexual repertoire.

"For me, there is a pleasure in physical intimacy and feeling connected to your partner," Kerry shared, "rather than feeling like you are both beginning some course of action that has to keep going until one or the other of you, or maybe both, but rarely at the same time, reaches some sexual milestone after which you are allowed to stop." She continued, "Without the feeling of 'I have to orgasm' or 'I have to make my partner orgasm,' we are free to focus on the joy of making the other person happy. Touching sensitive spots like genitals, nipples and other parts just feels good. Besides, sex should be play and it should be fun." Kerry, you nailed it!

Women can still enjoy sex without orgasm. Around 10 to 15 percent of women cannot/do not orgasm at all, and around 1–5 percent of men are anorgasmic. If this is you, it's totally okay if you are okay with it; however, your inability to orgasm (or for your partner to do so) may have a medical cause, such as diabetes or multiple sclerosis, so be sure these diagnoses are ruled out by your doctor.

Let's take the focus off what isn't happening and focus on what is. Feeling sexually lame because you have never orgasmed is denying yourself the right to define sexual pleasure for yourself. I am calling bullshit on orgasm as the litmus test of sexual proficiency. This sexual measuring stick was created by men centuries ago, who lived when women were property, essentially to be used by men for procreation and pleasure.

But now, in the wake of menopause awareness, female sexual pleasure has begun to germinate as a concept and the female orgasm as a sexual norm has gone from perhaps to possible, an objective stamp of gendered sexual equality. A cautionary note: While orgasmic equality might seem a feminist milestone worth striving for, if we aim for mandatory female orgasm as a prerequisite for gender-balanced sex, we set ourselves up for yet another version of performance anxiety. A healthier approach is to view good sex as whatever brings you *pleasure* rather than whatever leads to orgasm. Orgasm equality in my opinion should not refract the female sexual experience through the lens of male sexual pleasure.

Causes of Impaired Ability or Inability to Orgasm

- Illicit or prescription drug use
- Alcohol use
- Diabetes
- Multiple sclerosis
- Depression medications: antidepressants, especially at a high dose
- Oral contraceptives

Let's make our own rules about what constitutes great sex, and let's not copy men or even each other on this point. Drink the wine you enjoy, not what someone else tells you to drink. Have the sex *you* want; not what other people tell you is good. That, my friends, is how we close the Bedroom Gap.

Chapter 7

The Five *M*'s

Patricia is looking down when I enter the room, her body posture defeated. "I don't know why I'm here," she says. "I don't even want to be here." I wait, knowing she needs time to convince herself to go on.

"I feel bad for him, for my husband," she continues. "There's nothing wrong with him. But he wants sex all the time. Well, not really all the time, but it seems like all the time. And I don't. I really *really* don't. Want sex, that is."

Versions of this scenario play out in my clinic all day long. I do a lot of listening. It takes women a long time to get in to see me, and they have usually waited a long time before getting up the nerve to even make the appointment. There is, sometimes, a reluctance, a dissonance, an inner turmoil, a conflicted feeling in the room with us. They are here to fix a problem, find a solution, please a partner. They are not always here at their own behest. And many of these women do not want to be here at all. They know there is a Bedroom Gap in their lives even if they don't know the term yet. Some want to close it—these women are hopeful that I will have a magic medication that will fix everything. Others hope there is no solution and that I will give them permission to continue to avoid sex. Many think closing the Bedroom Gap will be good for their marriage, but very few realize or dare to hope that closing this gap might be exciting and rejuvenating *for them*.

But if you're reading these pages, you might be ready by now to think carefully about how beneficial it might be to close the Bedroom Gap for yourself.

Now that we know that the Bedroom Gap exists—and here you are in my virtual office, willing to consider some help—it's time for us to discuss the various methods you can use to close your own gap. I call these hot tips the Five *M*'s, and my patients love them. We will also talk about some other resources you can use on your own or with a therapist.

What are the Five *M*'s? They are:

1. Mindfulness
2. Massage
3. Masturbation
4. Media
5. Medications

Before I can tell patients about the five *M*'s, I need to get a bit of history from them. What's your history, what's your partner's history, and what is your shared history? Also, what history and, in some cases, baggage, did each of you bring to the bedroom?

You might begin with your own version of Patricia's story, something along the lines of: We have been married thirty years (or twenty, or ten, or two), but we used to have more sex. Yes, the sex was fine, sometimes even great, but now I don't want to have sex. And my partner does. Really does. And it is affecting our relationship.

Try This Sex Therapy Kick Start

If you are lucky enough to find a professional someone to work with you on improving your sex life, **here are some questions you can answer and even preemptively share with your clinician or counselor to help get things going**:

1. I learned about sex from _____

2. The messages about sex as I was growing up were
   - _____ from my mother
   - _____ from my father
   - _____ from siblings, friends

3. My first sexual experience went like this:

4. I have a history of (circle any or none): nonconsensual sex/childhood sexual trauma/sexual assault/rape

5. I gender identify as:

6. I describe my sexual interests as:

7. My current partner is: (name, age, his/her/their relevant medical or sexual history). Are you monogamous? Has there been infidelity? Are you attracted to him/her/them? Do you feel it is reciprocal attraction?

8. Do you masturbate/have you ever masturbated? What words come to mind when you hear the word *masturbation*?

9. How do you feel about pornography? What words come to mind when you hear the word *porn*?

10. How I feel about my body right now:

11. How I feel about sex right now:

12. I orgasm never/rarely/sometimes/often/always

13. I orgasm from clitoral stimulation/vaginal stimulation/both

14. Orgasm itself is important to me: y/n

15. How has sex changed for you as you've gotten older?

16. I want to improve my sex life because _____

Once I get some of the background from them, I ask my patients to share what they learned about sex from (1) their parents, (2) their friends/youth/first partner/past partners, and (3) from their current partner. Some questions I ask include: Was sex talked about at home? Was it a shameful topic? Where did that shame come from? Was there ever a relative with a teen pregnancy? Did you learn about sex in school? Was this topic ever dinner table talk? Was masturbation frowned upon? Was it implicitly sanctioned for boys but not girls? Were there different gendered standards in the family with respect to sex as an entitlement, or a goal, or a source of braggadocio?

Often the answers to these questions give color and offer clues as to what is going on in your own bedroom, where we have work to do, and how we might approach improving the sexual experience.

Almost no matter how the questions are answered, using the five *M*'s improves the quality and sometimes quantity of sex that is happening. Let's dig in.

M-1: Mindfulness

Having trouble keeping stress or your past or future issues out of the bedroom? This section is for you. Mindfulness can help you be there, in the bedroom, in the moment.

When a woman comes to see me for sexual counseling, we eventually get to the chocolate bar appointment. We sit in comfortable chairs and do the exercise together. (No way am I going to watch my patient eat chocolate without getting some for myself!)

What does the chocolate bar exercise involve? We sit together and very, very slowly take in the bar: its size, weight, shape. The feel of the wrapper, the design of the art, the font, the colors. Is the lettering raised? Embossed? Calligraphic? Then we slide the paper cover off slowly. We look at the glossy metallic wrapper. Now there's only one layer between our fingertips and the chocolate. We open the foil wrapper methodically (or tear it open—dealer's choice). We smell the aroma. We do everything but taste the chocolate until we've really taken in all the multisensory information on sight, feel, sound, and smell that we can. Only then do we break off some chocolate and place it in our mouths. Maybe. Some patients just savor what they experienced and save the chocolate for later.

This, my friends, is mindfulness—paying attention to every detail of the present moment, to increase the pleasure you might feel during it. Mindfulness is known to decrease stress and help manage anxiety, not just in sexual situations, but in life!

I want to cover a few specific approaches to mindfulness here that might help you in the bedroom.

Mindfulness-Based Stress Reduction (MBSR)

The first is mindfulness-based stress reduction (MBSR). Based on the mindfulness meditation work of Dr. Jon Kabat-Zinn, MBSR is the simple practice of, in Kabat-Zinn's own words, "awareness that arises through paying attention, on purpose, in the present moment, non-judgmentally . . . in the service of self-understanding and wisdom."[1] MBSR has been shown to help with stress reduction and menopausal symptoms and can even help patients cope with a variety of illnesses.

Let's try it out with a short meditation. Yes, right now. It'll just take a minute and then we can get back to talking about sex.

What are you thinking about right now? Is the grass getting scraggly on your lawn? Have you still not dropped off your dry cleaning? Are you hyper-focused on eating the remaining half of that carrot muffin on the kitchen counter? Take those thoughts and "watch" them as if at a distance, as if they are blades of grass swirling and floating on the surface of a stream or river. Allow them to pass you by and keep going down that river.

You can start these brief practices alone, but you can also do this with your partner right next to you, whether that partner is awake or asleep. Kabat-Zinn suggests we be aware of the "feeling of the human next to you, whether you have known that human for sixty years or sixty seconds."[2]

This struck me as being totally applicable to connecting with your partner in the bedroom. How many of us habitually climb into bed with a boatload of issues or worries about impending ones, either to fall asleep (or not) or to reflexively give in to sex without being fully appreciative of the human we spend hours next to?

Pause. Appreciate the totality of the moment as you are lying there, and of the person next to you and what it means to be there with that person in that moment. It is small, just a moment, but it is significant if you let it be so.

Now that your head is a bit clearer, try to focus on just being in the present moment. Right here, right now. What do you want to focus on? The book you've been wanting to read. The difficult sympathy card you want to write for your friend who lost her father last week. What if you try to focus on spontaneous or scheduled time to work on intimacy with your partner? Not sex, mind you, but just being alone together with a clear mind. If you are telling yourself right now that you lack the time or you just can't add mindfulness for intimacy to your routine, I would urge you to make the time, to show up for it as if it were a recurring work or social event on your Google calendar.

Mindfulness can take place for two minutes when you wake and two minutes as you climb into bed; you don't need incense and a ringing bowl, just an awareness and intentionality about life moments, including sexual moments. Kabat-Zinn may be the OG but also check out Dr. Lori Brotto's eight-week, mindfulness-based sex therapy course at Brottolab.com; her course teaches MBSR techniques with the aim of improved sexual focus.

Mindfulness practice can even affect your relationship with food. Mindful eating, the basis of the chocolate bar experience above, involves embracing food as a multisensory experience: Slowly, deliberately putting a fork down between bites to focus on the flavors and textures of the food in your mouth. Tasting the five flavor essences: sweet, sour, salty, savory (or umami), and bitter—and letting yourself appreciate the tastes and how they change as you chew the food. How does the food smell? How does the taste echo or contradict the smell?

How about the texture of the food—the snap of truly crispy bacon or a perfect baguette, a flaky croissant, the juicy bite of a crisp apple, or the crunch of a carrot? The tannic flavors of a good cabernet sauvignon, the somewhat gritty crystals of really good Parmesan, the umami flavor of soy sauce or green tea? Trust me, if you can eat mindfully, you can be mindful in other areas too.

If you really think about mindfulness in terms of attention to sex, you appreciate your own body and that of your partner on a whole new level. The curve of a hip, the responsiveness of a nipple, the familiarity of a birthmark—anything can be a part of a sexual mindfulness that personalizes and enhances your sexual experience.

Cognitive Behavioral Therapy (CBT)

The second method of mindfulness-based stress management is cognitive behavioral therapy (CBT)—a blend of behavioral and cognitive actions taken together. The goal is to elicit a "relaxation response," which will in turn reduce stress, anxiety, and fear. Yoga and hypnosis can also elicit this response. Find what clicks for you.

CBT involves identifying irrational thought patterns and questioning their validity by addressing and challenging those irrational thoughts, then reframing them with more natural ways of thinking. For example: Am I likely to get AIDS by having sex with a partner after an affair even if he has shown me negative testing? Or, if I have sex, will it cause the abnormal cells from my breast cancer to spread? The rational answer to both of these questions is no, but irrational fears are hard to shed.

CBT also includes techniques to reduce stress, such as diaphragmatic breathing exercises and progressive muscle relaxation.[3] How does this apply to sex? Well, if you're anticipating sexual pain, you can preemptively do deep breathing exercises, after which you can identify, tighten, and then relax muscle groups such as gluteal muscles, leg muscles, neck and jaw and pelvic floor muscles (think Kegels) *before sex* to help you locate what is reflexively tightening during foreplay or prior to or during insertion. This way, you can notice the muscles tightening in response to anticipatory anxiety and actively relax them.

Using vaginal trainers, also called vaginal dilators, or a vibrator can help you do this as well. You can feel the tension when inserting a dilator and intentionally relax around it. Pelvic Floor Physical Therapists are specially trained to help with sexual pain among other things. We will learn more about this type of therapy in the next section.

If mindfulness seems a bit too woo-woo to actually be helpful, or even necessary, in the bedroom, think again. Women who dread sex are not uncommon. In fact, 6 to 16 percent of women have stress related to anticipation of sex.[4] The World Health Organization listed the current global population of women of reproductive age at 1.9 billion.[5] Now add the 1 billion menopausal-age women, and you have nearly 3 billion women globally who are potentially sexually active. If even just 10 percent of those women have stress related to the anticipation of sex, that is three hundred million women dreading sex, whether the cause is fear of pain or STI or pregnancy or just sexual dread from past life events.

To make matters worse, I would venture to say the prevalence of vaginismus, pain with sex, and sexual trauma are vastly underreported. Recall that two hundred million women worldwide are victims of female genital mutilation, which carries both PTSD-level trauma and often unbearable pain with sex. These numbers are also likely underreported, so you can imagine how enormous the figures are if we were to accurately include all women for whom sex is anxiety provoking.

Whether it's pain, trauma, or just general anxiety, it's all part of the shame women feel when they buy into the media images of women enjoying sex. They can't help but think, *Why can't I be more like that? Why does it seem like every other woman is enjoying sex but not me?* Too many women feel broken, alone, atypical, but most are very reluctant to share those issues with friends or clinicians.

The number of women who enter a bedroom with anxiety and fear—regardless of the reason why—is not small. Even if your own anxiety and fear stems from a non-sex-related place, say a recent childbirth, surgery, or bicycle accident, you can benefit from the stress reduction techniques we are talking about here.

The key point is that we need to learn to pay attention to where our fear and anxiety surrounding sex is coming from. Sometimes a CBT-trained therapist or mindfulness-based stress reduction course can help us connect the dots and liberate us from the irrational thinking that leads to fears and aversions in the bedroom.

Pelvic Floor Physical Therapy (PFPT)

The physical therapy counterpart to MBSR and CBT is pelvic floor physical therapy (PFPT), a type of physical therapy that focuses on releasing tension in muscles and ligaments in the pelvis. This might not sound like it fits in the mindfulness section of the 5Ms, but in fact it does. A pelvic floor physical therapist can teach you relaxation techniques—see, mindfulness!—and help you reduce sexual pain using breathing techniques, exercises, dilators, and other devices.

For example, as we discussed earlier, a therapist can work with you on being conscious of the tension you feel when inserting a device and teach you ways to relax, acknowledging the fear and learning to master it, and teach your muscles to respond in kind.[6] It is beyond the scope of this book to go into the amazing ways a PFPT can help you with an awareness of your pelvic floor, including improvement in bowel and bladder control, reduction in pelvic pain, and recovery from childbirth or injury. But if you have anticipatory anxiety around sex, consider PFPT as a physical counterpart and/or adjunct therapy to CBT and MBSR.

Try This: Putting Your Training into Practice, Starting with G-Rated Touching

You and your partner can begin to practice sexual mindfulness together before moving on to the second *M*, massage. All the mindfulness training you've just done will help you focus on observing sensations in your body.

To start moving into the more physical realm of mindfulness, try scheduling a weekly thirty-minute hangout date with your partner. This isn't a sex date! No sex at all, in fact; I just want you to clear your schedule for togetherness. Once a couple is doing this regularly, you can add in mindfulness-based touching but only in a "G-rated way." This means touching parts of the body not typically associated with sexual arousal. Avoid the genitals, nipples, lips, even the earlobes . . . for now. Focus elsewhere intentionally and touch each other only when you want to. Notice the sensations of receiving touch from your partner and also how it feels to be the partner doing the touching.

After some time trying this out, expand the touching exercise to sexually sensitive areas. Again, be aware of how you feel while you are being touched and when you are doing the touching. Be aware of your breathing, of how relaxed you are. If your thoughts drift to the laundry or your to-do list, acknowledge that, then imagine the to-do list floating like a paper on the same swirling river as the blades of grass we imagined before, and let it travel away. Then focus your thoughts back on the touch or smell or taste or sight of what you're doing. Remember, you don't have to have any starting baseline sexual desire to do this exercise. Often sexual interest develops from the effort. But don't worry if it doesn't—just notice what you *are* feeling in the moment and enjoy any and all sensations you feel without attaching any expectations to those feelings.

No partner? No problem. Mindfulness works for masturbation, certainly, but also for nonsexual activities, such as walks in nature, having a warm mug of tea on your couch, or any other solo activity you can think of. Even making the time for a long, decadent bath, being aware of the scents, the sound of the water, and the joy of luxuriating in the solitude of the moment can be more gratifying if done mindfully.

M-2: Massage

Now that you have a foundation for understanding the importance of being in the moment, of the *intentionality* of the moments you are devoting to how your body feels, to feeling connected, to being open to intimacy and maybe even to sex, let's move from the first M to the second and focus on one of the more powerful tools to light up the erotic receptive parts of your brain: touch.

Whether experiencing pleasure from touching your own body or touching another human, we know that touch can lead to sexual arousal by generating pleasure. Specifically, the skin's nerve endings carry information to areas of the brain that process the sensation, release hormones, and generate emotion. Touch can trigger the release of oxytocin, which, remember, we learned is a "bonding" hormone. Oxytocin also inhibits the stress response. Touch can also lead to dopamine release, which tells us that touch is rewarding. Slow, gentle stroking in particular triggers a response in specific nerve endings, which pass on signals to the areas of the brain that control emotion, reward, and pleasurable sensations.[7]

Massage can be an informal version of repetitive touching of your partner, or it can be intentionally sensual or sexual. Sexual massage is massage with the intention of leading to a sexual experience. Types of sexual massage include tantric massage and nuru. Tantric massage involves deep breathing and the slow massage of erogenous zones. One of the aims of tantric massage is to promote spiritual growth and connectivity between the recipient and massagist. The objective is the giving and receiving of pleasure without orgasm expectation.

Nuru massage is full body contact with both partners coated in oil or gel. This massage technique originated in Japan and has been practiced for pay in massage parlors, and although it might sound a bit messy to try at home, it doesn't mean you can't adapt some amount of slipperiness and fun to your own private version of massage.

M-3: **Masturbation**

Masturbation might feel like a bit of a taboo subject to some people, but I am here to remind you that the practice is neither shocking nor shameful, and it is certainly nothing new. It is an activity that has been traced back in human history forty million years and also occurs throughout the entire animal kingdom.[8] In humans, the general acceptance of masturbation as a justifiable behavior has had a rocky road, from tacit acceptance as a sexual outlet for high libido to disdain bordering on disgust for an aberrant pathological behavior. As the behavioral scientist Thomas Szasz put it, "in the nineteenth century it was a disease. In the twentieth, it's a cure."[9]

However history feels about it, the word, the image, the concept is so unsettling to many of my patients and some of my friends that it is one of the hardest things we discuss together. And yet, if you simply think of masturbation as a version of touching your own body to elicit pleasure, it isn't really that scary.

Perhaps some of the awkward scariness comes from the idea of masturbation being only about one thing, a designated objective: an orgasm. It can be intimidating to begin to do something without really ever being told how, not to mention believing you had to do it so well that you achieved the goal of orgasm. Can you imagine skiing without knowledge of how to put on the boots, use the poles, the bindings, the skis, or the chairlift? While also being told that at the end of the run you need to be flying off a very high ski jump, or else you've failed? No wonder masturbation freaks some people out!

Hollywood hasn't helped. Too many women have been portrayed as orgasming in under thirty seconds from mostly clothed, missionary, stand-up sex while pushed up against a jukebox. Perhaps some women can pull that off, but most of us wouldn't come close to orgasming in those circumstances.

Sure, things might be a little easier when you're alone, but the pressure to "achieve" an orgasm by yourself is still there. To make matters worse, since many women have historically been encouraged not to touch themselves as girls or young women, there is a reluctance at a deep psychological level even to contemplate masturbation. We are in some way disobeying our mothers or Sunday school teachers or aunts or someone who led us to believe that masturbation was dirty or forbidden. For others there is simply an anatomic challenge of not really knowing what is where, or even what feels good!

How do I masturbate? Here are some basics I share with patients, with a nod of thanks to Emily Nagoski.[10]

1. **Make some private time.** Even fifteen to thirty minutes. Absolutely shed any form of disruption or distraction (TV, smartphone, smartwatch, etc.) and make the setting relaxing. Maybe that means you're playing music that makes you feel calm. Maybe lighting a candle helps release your stress. Create whatever setting you need to feel at ease.

2. **Know or get to know your anatomy.** If you haven't done so already, take out a mirror and start getting to know your parts.

3. **Start G-rated.** Touch your arms, legs, hands, wrists, feet, ankles, tummy, neck. Anywhere that your brain tells your hands it feels nice to touch, then touch that. Try different speeds of strokes, and different sensations. Fingertips, fingernails, with lotion or oil, or without. You might just stick with G-rated touching for the first several times you do this. It feels great, doesn't cost anything, and also helps you learn what you like, and what you might want to tell a partner you like.

4. **Progress to PG-rated.** Touch your upper inner thighs, breasts, and other areas that are somewhat erogenous; repeat this as many sessions as feels comfortable before you progress further.

5. When you feel ready, **touch your Mons Pubis**, the soft puffy part of your vulva where there is (or was) hair, above and on the pubic bone. Light or firm direct pressure, or round or rocking motion of your palm on the Mons is a simple way to start.

6. Now try tugging or pressing or **stimulating the labia**; add some warm lube or an oil if it suits you.

7. Try directly touching **the clitoris itself**, in different ways, with different motions and pressures until you find what you like. For some women, they only touch the clitoris after they are fairly aroused with indirect stimulation, or they only stimulate the clitoris with a vibrator or a tub faucet or shower head. Experiment and decide what you like.

8. **Orgasm is not the goal**, but it can be an outcome. Don't try to make yourself orgasm. Give yourself permission to allow pleasure to take whatever form at whatever level it occurs.

9. **Enjoy** what you are doing, and if you are frustrated or something doesn't feel great, stop, go back to what you were doing that did feel good and build from there.

M-4: Media

Media is the easiest, and the hardest, of the five *M*'s. Easy because media is so easily and inexpensively accessible to anyone with a smartphone. Hard because as soon as I say the word *porn*, or adult film, some women put their hand up and stop me. "No thanks," they say, "that stuff is not my cup of tea." Or worse, "How can you, as a gynecologist and advocate for women, mention something so degrading to our gender?"

But when I say media, I'm not just talking about the porn you (don't want to) watch. Today we can get sexually informed and stimulated through many media forms, from podcasts to audio porn. The female brain benefits from erotic stimulation whether visual (TV and film), auditory (erotic stories), or written (erotic literature). We store the sights, sounds, and stories and they keep our brains primed for intimacy. Good news: There is so much out there. You just have to find the media to consume that strikes the right chord with your sexual juju. Check out the suggestions in the "Podcasts and Porn Sites, Oh My" appendix.

M-5 Medications

Are there medications that can help close the Bedroom Gap? Yes, with a few caveats. They work but not for everybody, not all the time, and not without side effects for some users. But since we do have them, and they are effective in some situations and for some people, you should at least be aware of your options.

Sometimes, when my patients have gone without sex for a long time and can't envision ever returning to the bedroom for sex itself, I use medications to kick the "no sex ever again" door down. Medication therapy cannot fix everything going wrong in your bedroom, but it can fill an ongoing neurochemical need or just kick-start a sleepy sex drive. Let's check them out.

Addyi
We talked about flibanserin, whose brand name is Addyi, in Chapter 2. If you recall, it was the first medication FDA-approved for female sexual health. For now, it is approved only for premenopausal women diagnosed with Hypoactive Sexual Desire Disorder (HSDD), or what non-clinicians simply call low libido.

Hypoactive Sexual Desire Disorder

HSDD, which affects (at least) 10 percent of US women, is defined as "persistent or recurrent absence of sexual fantasies and desire for sexual activity, causing marked personal distress or interpersonal difficulties, which must be present for at least six months."[11] HSDD is more prevalent in partnered and sexually inactive women and the peak age is 40–64.

HSDD can be diagnosed by you or any clinician with five easy questions from the Decreased Sexual Desire Screener (DSDS).[12] If someone wants to know if they "qualify" as having low desire, here are the five questions:

1. In the past, was your level of sexual desire or interest good and satisfying to you? Y/N
2. Has there been a decrease in your level of sexual desire or interest? Y/N
3. Are you bothered by your decreased level of sexual desire or interest? Y/N
4. Would you like your level of sexual desire or interest to increase? Y/N
5. Do any of the following factors contribute to your current decrease in sexual desire or interest?
    a. Surgery, injuries, depression, or other medical condition
    b. Medications, drugs, or alcohol you are currently taking/ using
    c. Pregnancy, recent childbirth, menopause
    d. Other sexual issues such as pain, decreased arousal, or decreased orgasm
    e. Your partner's sexual problems
    f. Dissatisfaction with your relationship or partner
    g. Stress or fatigue

If you answered yes to the first four and no to question 5, then you qualify as having generalized, acquired HSDD and may benefit from one of the medications discussed here.

We don't know precisely how Addyi works in the brain, but it likely promotes secretion of dopamine and norepinephrine, which in turn increases desire. Just like SSRIs and SNRIs for depression, it takes about a month before you may notice its effects.

If you are interested in getting started with Addyi, I recommend trying it for two months, perhaps three, before deciding whether it works for you. The most common side effects are sleepiness, loss of appetite, and nausea. Take Addyi at bedtime to minimize your awareness of these side effects. Addyi taken with alcohol can cause a drop in blood pressure, so skip your evening dose of the medicine if you have consumed more than two standard drinks (two beers, two glasses of wine, two shots of hard alcohol) within two hours of when you usually take Addyi. (If unsure, just skip your dose. Easy.)

Addyi is actually a very safe and very easy medication to try. If, after two to three months, you don't notice any nudge forward in your sexual interest, or any increase in your satisfaction around the sex you are having, you can stop Addyi without needing to wean or taper off. It is one dose fits all.

Vyleesi

Bremelanotide, whose brand name is Vyleesi, was also mentioned in Chapter 2; it is the first and only on-demand medication to be FDA approved for low sex drive in (premenopausal) women and the second medication to be FDA-approved for HSDD.

How does it work? Bremelanotide mimics certain neurotransmitters in the brain, selectively turning on receptors that result in a dopamine release leading to an intense feeling of wanting to have sex.[13] Women taking it love that it is on demand, more akin to how their partners might use an ED med like Viagra, and that they don't have to take something like Addyi every day just to have sex a few times a month.

My patients sometimes use it when they have a holiday planned with their partner. One patient, June, and her husband, Ray, have quarterly getaways to escape their busy professional and family lives. "We usually just rent an AirBnB or hotel, but once a year we go on a cruise," June tells me. She uses Vyleesi for these getaways because she wants to be sure that when they have the opportunity to have sex, that she is eager and "in the mood." "Vyleesi is my security blanket, my secret weapon," she confides. "It's my injectable sex drive, and it doesn't disappoint."

Sounds amazing, right? Well, like many things that seem too good to be true, Vyleesi has some down sides. Nausea is a problem but usually only with the first injection. It lasts about two hours and decreases or is absent after subsequent injections. I suggest that the first time you try Vyleesi, your only sex partner be a vibrator and a video and that you have no expectations for sex that night in case your nausea is severe or prolonged. Your second injection should be intended to be the real deal, though. You should inject Vyleesi into the abdomen or thigh about forty-five minutes before you want to get your sex game on. The package insert recommends against more than one dose within twenty-four hours and also suggests no more than eight doses per month because of the 1 percent risk of focal hyperpigmentation on the face, gums, or nipples. High cost and poor insurance coverage limit the number of women who can splurge on this box of injectable lust. But those who can afford it and don't mind the side effects describe an "incredible rush, almost like the high from illegal drugs." Because the feeling lasts for twelve to fifteen hours, women who use it sometimes have evening sex, then wake up and want more sex.

Testosterone: At Last, and Not Yet

As researchers continue to uncover the chemistry of female sexual desire, there has been a medical therapy hiding in plain sight: testosterone, or T for short.

As we learned earlier, women make testosterone and men make estrogen. It's true. Every single woman on the planet makes T, and women of every age rely on it as a source to create estrogen, as a contributor to sex drive, and also to keep our bones strong, our muscles developed, and our brains alight. But like estrogen, testosterone made in the ovaries decreases after menopause.

Testosterone can and should be part of menopausal hormone therapy (HT), and there should be FDA-approved formulations available to ensure stable and predictable dosing for women. There are more than thirty FDA-approved T therapies for men and zero for women. Zero. Yikes. Another biopharma and FDA–created contribution to the Bedroom Gap if ever there was one.

But there are solutions to this oversight! Here are three ways the FDA can move the T needle forward so that everybody, every female body that is, who would benefit from T can get it safely and maybe even get it covered by insurance, just like men do. First, think about how menopause is a hormone deficiency state that affects 100 percent of humans with ovaries; that deficiency includes testosterone, which is made in the ovaries at four times the amount as estrogen. Why not include testosterone as a medical need akin to estrogen and progesterone to address health issues for all women who lose ovarian steroids whether from menopause or other causes? T is FDA approved for men with hypogonadism and low T. Why not extend women the same courtesy? Second, address how T is classified. It is a Schedule III controlled substance, classified as such due to its potential for misuse, abuse, and dependency as an anabolic steroid. This is from an outdated 1990 law that was created in response to an Olympic doping scandal. Get T removed from the DEA's list of dangerous drugs. This will free up the ability to prescribe T more easily, thus enabling women to get T if they live in an area without a menopause trained clinician. Third, look at the data we have and fund the data we need to get an FDA-approved formulation. As I write this, the only options for women are to get it compounded at pharmacies in topical creams or to use one tenth of the dose of male formulation. Neither option is covered nor easy to obtain. One promising idea is that in June 2025 the FDA announced a program to accelerate drug reviews for products that align with US Health priorities and enhance health interests of Americans. The product must address an unmet public health need (check) and should be an innovative or first-in-class approach to treatment (check). Why not put testosterone on the fast-track approval it deserves?

Is testosterone for you, and is it safe? Yes, and yes. But don't take it from me. There is a global consensus among leading clinicians who study hormonal therapy regarding use of testosterone for women. In 2019 they published the "Global Consensus Position Statement on the Use of Testosterone Therapy for Women."[14] The statement's key takeaways (and my thoughts in italics) include:

- Testosterone therapy is the only evidence-based treatment for hypoactive sexual desire disorder (HSDD) in *post*menopausal women.
- Testosterone therapy can improve many facets of sexual function, including desire, arousal, orgasm, and pleasure, and reduce stress and distress related to sex. *And don't forget it likely impacts bone, brain, musculoskeletal health, and genital health in a positive way.*
- Testosterone therapy, especially at high doses, can have side effects. *These include acne, increased facial and/or body hair, weight gain, male pattern baldness, elevation in blood pressure, elevation in LDL "bad" cholesterol, reduction in HDL "good" cholesterol, type 2 diabetes, blood clots in the lungs*

or deep veins; pelvic pain, discomfort in the clitoris, making too many red blood cells, called polycythemia, and changes in mood. Side effects are more likely if given orally or in high doses, such as with T pellets. Anecdotally, I have been using low dose topical testosterone for women for many years with minimal side effects; given transdermally at a low dose I find it very safe and easy to use.

- Meta-analyses of studies show an excellent short-term safety profile of testosterone in physiologic doses. *This means the results of many studies pooled together show that if testosterone is given to women to restore their testosterone levels to within a normal premenopausal range, it is safe, at least in the short term.*

- We do not have adequate long-term safety studies on exogenous testosterone use in women. *We need large, randomized, placebo-controlled studies, and we need funding for said studies. Biotech investors, scientific investigators, FDA commissions, wake up! That said, we are not starting from zero. Gender-affirming hormone therapy (GAHT) in transmasculine people did not show any dangerous side effects to testosterone therapy. And let me share from a conversation with my fellow testosterone-obsessed colleague, Dr. Kelly Casperson:[15] "We always say there are no long-term safety studies for women with respect to testosterone. But we have given trans men doses of testosterone at 10 times the normal testosterone levels of women and have been doing this for 30 years and have followed these patients and have seen no evidence of increases in heart disease or cancers or other dangerous effects; they do have androgenic effects such as oily skin, acne and hair growth, but in the case of the trans men, they chose to take the T because they wanted hair growth. And remember, the doses were 10 times the dose that we would give for women who just want to close the gap of hormone deficiency, including testosterone deficiency from menopause. Think about it. How many drugs have to be dosed at 10 times the physiologic range and studied long term to pass muster at the FDA? None." Thank you, Kelly, you wise soul.*

What study data do we have today to support the safety and usefulness of T therapy in women?

- An article reviewing the safety of testosterone therapy from 8,000+ women in the UK *showed no increased risk of breast cancer, hepatitis, cardiovascular disease, diabetes, or blood clots.*[16]
- Safety data from articles published between 1980 and 2010—over thirty years—focused on low dose testosterone therapy for transsexuals, which reported *no increased risk of mortality, breast cancer, or vascular disease.*[17]
- Available testosterone therapies for women include intramuscular and subcutaneous injections and transdermal gels and creams as well as implantable pellets.

There are lots of ways you can give your brain and body a small, female level of testosterone to make up for the menopausal testosterone deficit. Any woman with signs or symptoms of testosterone deficiency such as reduced libido is a candidate for topical testosterone therapy. If your clinician is unaware or uncomfortable prescribing testosterone for you, find one who is, and help your libido safely and easily.

So far, we have learned about the biological basis of sex—about our anatomy, about desire, and about pleasure. We have learned about how the rocket blast launch of Viagra widened the Bedroom Gap for many midlife couples, making the sexual playing field even more uneven. And we have learned some strategies—the five *M*'s—for starting to close your own Bedroom Gap at home.

Now, in Part 3, we will learn about the education that needs to happen on both an individual and a societal, even global, scale. From the reframing of sex ed for teens to the renovation of the medical education system to the overhaul of how we access clinical care, this section will tackle some of the really big things that have happened and still need to happen if we are to address the Bedroom Gap as a global gender issue. Let's start with overhauling menopause and sex education.

PART THREE

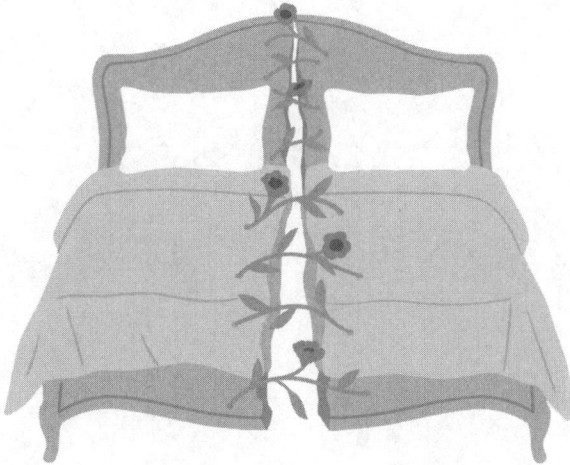

Chapter 8

Repositioning Sex Ed

If we're going to close the Bedroom Gap on a big, collective level, it's imperative that we talk about what society can do better on our behalf. I want to point the education spotlight on two areas that desperately need reimagining: sex ed for teens and sex ed for clinicians. If we can improve how we learn about sex early on, we, the sexual consumer, are more likely to have agency over our sexual choices and outcomes. If we can improve how educated and comfortable clinicians are in talking about sexual health, they can more readily receive our issues and offer helpful guidance.

Revamping Sex Ed for Teens

Actor and menopause advocate Naomi Watts recently described perimenopause and menopause as "the adult version of puberty—this is puberty in reverse. I wish that this [education about menopause] would happen in Sex Ed in fifth grade. It's just part of it, and for some reason, that part of the story was just left out."[1]

In Naomi Watts's dream world redux, and mine as well, sex ed in school would explain that women have *two* milestones in terms of their reproductive health—puberty and perimenopause. Both are hormonally chaotic periods when bodies and brains change dramatically. But no high school sex ed class previews the hormonal double whammy of puberty and perimenopause for those born with two X chromosomes. Nor do they teach kids about what happens to men. They might learn about how their testosterone levels explode between ages ten and eighteen, but very few people learn about *what happens as men age*, to their bodies and their sexual health. It should come as no surprise then that such hormonal shifts often surprise or confound us.

"The book end of puberty," as Watts has referred to it, is waiting for every single one of us women. And we need to take it upon ourselves to get educated about what this means rather than waiting for doctors to tell us what is going on.

Watts herself had the rude awakening that she was perimenopausal at age thirty-six when she was trying to get pregnant and her blood tests showed she was "heading towards menopause." "My mom was 45 when she became menopausal and I didn't realize there was a whole decade before that of symptoms and issues," she says.[2]

Or take the very public story of Tamsen Fadel, an Emmy-award winning journalist and TV newscaster who experienced a hot flash while filming a news segment and was completely dumbfounded as to what was going on. "It was November 2019, and I was in the news studio and I had a really significant hot flash, you know the kind where your heart is racing, and you feel really sick and you don't know whether you're gonna throw up or pass out. You just don't know what's happening. I didn't want to be an alarmist, and I was in a studio full of guys, but I also didn't want to pass out on the air. I thought my story was unique and came to find out it was anything but."[3]

Why is it that so many women are surprised about menopause and perimenopause? How could something so universal, so ubiquitous in a woman's lifespan, be left out of the conversation, whether between mother and daughter, or sex ed/human development class, or the doctor's office? Perhaps menopause and andropause are chronologically too far off to merit inclusion in the curricula of middle school sex ed classes, or maybe this is further evidence of the ageism and sexism in health care. But I would venture to say that the outdated, gender-slanted, ageist content of present-day sex ed classes has set us up for midlife ignorance and confusion about how our bodies age, including sexually. If sex ed classes neglect to teach you about the sexual function of male and female bodies *across their lifespan*, of course you won't know what to expect and will be left completely befuddled when you experience peri/menopause symptoms.

The pleasure-deficient aspect of sex education causes other problems too. This is a big and important point. If sex ed doesn't include teaching about pleasure and desire, how will we be equipped to *prioritize pleasure in our earliest sexual relationships* and to *keep this a priority even when the sexual function of our bodies changes with age*? If you are not taught early, or at all, about the more nuanced aspects of sex such as pleasure and desire, you are further set up to struggle, sexually speaking, as the mechanics of sex change with age and come up short in your ability to have a gratifying sexual experience for yourself and for your partner.

Sex Ed Today

Kristi is a member of her school's Teen Peer Education Program, called Teen PEP, a popular club at Princeton High School. Members are taught about sex education and then spend their school year educating their peers about sex and consent and pregnancy. What a great idea! Except that it usually fails, miserably.

Kristi herself came to see me during a free period in the fall of her junior year in high school. "I think I might be pregnant," she blurted out. "I had unprotected sex, then got my period the next day, and forgot to take my birth control pill before we had sex." This story is frustrating for me to hear. Kristi, a trained peer-to-peer sexual health educator, of all people should know exactly how things work in the contraception and safe sex department. First, she should be aware that having sex the day before your next cycle starts is not likely to culminate in pregnancy since women are only fertile for a few days of each cycle and are not fertile the day before a period starts.[4] Second, she knows (or so I thought) that unprotected sex is a setup both for STIs and unintended pregnancy, and that birth control pills are taken every day, not as some post-sex pregnancy prevention like some sort of sex-adjacent Tums. Did she not hear any of the lectures in Teen PEP? A tiny part of me worries that even the Teen PEP educator doesn't get it and is passing on myths and miseducation to the teens she is supposed to be training to be peer educators!

Teen Sex Ed Is in Trouble

Teen sex ed in the United States is in bad shape. Every year, girls like Kristi come into my clinic with situations and stories that reflect just how much they *aren't* being taught in sex ed class. They present to my clinic with unintended pregnancies, STIs, and confusion about how contraception works, about when they can get pregnant, and when they can't. They share tales of painful and often nonconsensual sexual encounters, sexual assaults, being roofied, same sex relationship issues, questions about vibrators, anal sex, and choking.[5] They feel embarrassment, confusion, shame. Some cling to the idea of the unbroken hymen as proof to their future spouse or their parents that they are virginal (see the text box on Virginity Is a Hoax). Why are teens and young adults so ill prepared for their sexual debut? How are so few ready for a successful if not enjoyable foray into sex? What's not working?

Virginity Is a Hoax

My colleague Dr. Faiza Sadiq, having fled the horrific regime of Saddam Hussein in Iraq, practiced gynecology on the back of a rusty truck in Yemen for nine years. Among her duties was to confirm "virginity tests" for families seeking to arrange marriages for daughters and nieces, often as young as eight years old. Dr. Faiza would pretend to examine the terrified girls and young women and always confirmed them as virgins, even when she suspected otherwise. "If I diagnosed them as non-virgins, they would be stoned or otherwise killed by their families, since that was the custom. Non-virgins brought shame to their families and had to be killed." Fantastic. Death as a punishment for loss of virginity. For a patriarchal construct.

But you thought virginity was a real thing, right? The diagnosis of virginity rests on the integrity of the hymen—a flimsy thin membrane covering the vaginal opening that gets destroyed with the first menstrual flow and then gets further broken apart with the use of tampons, vibrators, penises, anything that gets inserted into the vagina. Any woman who has menstruated does not have an "imperforate" or nonbroken hymen. *For clarification's sake, let me remind you that virginity is not a real thing.* Having sex for the first time is a real thing we can unpack at another time, but being labeled a virgin, or not, based on the integrity of a flimsy bit of membrane called a hymen is not a real thing. Not now. Not ever. What about blood-stained sheets with your first time having sex? Sixty percent of women don't bleed the first time they have PIV sex. Their hymen had long since been broken by menstrual flow, or by their riding a bike, using a tampon, or masturbating.

The most public instance of this Hymenal Hoax involved the careful inspection of the vaginal opening of then–Lady Diana Spencer by the Royal Gynecologist as a prerequisite for marriage to (the not virginal!) Prince Charles. This was less than fifty years ago. What did the gynecologist who "confirmed" her virginity find? Nothing. There was nothing to find because she had been menstruating (and probably masturbating and possibly having sex) for years, and so the vaginal opening was certainly not closed off. An intact hymen signified sexual purity, which is in theory what the Royal HooHa-ologist would have been looking to confirm. Was there some sort of royal minimum opening size the gynecologist was looking for? A certain ne'er been touched by a penis shape? What if Diana had used super plus tampons? Would she have failed the tiny untouched vagina test? Knowing that the global British Empire was waiting with bated breath to hear the results of his exam, and that she was already beloved in the public eye, how else could he answer but "Yes! The hymen is intact!" God Save the Queen!!

The Teen PEP curriculum at our local high school is, like many others across the country, rooted in preventing pregnancy and disease. The overarching tone of sex ed for teens throughout the United States *is fear-based rather than pleasure-based*. The messaging is, "Don't have sex or bad things will happen to you." Remember the "just don't have sex, don't do it!" scene in the movie *Mean Girls*? If you haven't seen it, look it up.[6] That movie came out over twenty years ago, and yet we are still getting it totally wrong!

Telling teens just not to have sex, or that to have sex is wrong and you will definitely get diseases and get pregnant if you *do* have sex, is not working. Teens want to have sex; their *bodies* badly want to have sex—they are all overflowing with hormones. They also think of sex as cool, mysterious, desirable, mature, and expected. Sex is something adults do, and they want to be the adult among their peers. They want to have sex to show they "got with" a girl, or a guy. Whether it is a sense of possession, accomplishment, romance, or bragging rights, teens think (a lot) about sex. There is strong pressure not only to have sex but to let your peers know you know *how* to have sex.

Sex education emphasizes wearing condoms to prevent disease and pregnancy. Okay, fine, except herpes and HPV, the two viruses responsible for a good amount of pathology, can still be transmitted even with a condom. Since condoms are prone to break, fall off, expire or be altogether forgotten, pregnancy prevention is better accomplished with a pill, patch, implant, or IUD. So why are we distilling sex ed down to avoiding pathology rather than promoting pleasure?

We teach a sanitized, heteronormative version of sex, aimed at the white middle class, which does not reflect the cultural, ethnic, and sexual heterogeneity of our times. This androcentric (male-focused) model of sex ed presumes ejaculation is the desired goal of sex, which means we've got to prevent pregnancy and disease transmission from that darn semen that is always, always looming in the forbidding sexual picture we are painting for young adults.

What if we started over? What if we scrapped the current curricula and built a sex ed platform from a standpoint whereby sex is not just a male-initiated, male-desired, male-driven act but one of mutual interest and initiative, where one outcome could be *pleasure for both partners*? Such pleasure-centered teaching would be inclusive to all gender identities, all pairings. Imagine if men were taught from high school to value female pleasure? How different might the Bedroom Gaps in midlife and throughout life be?

Pleasure Forward Sex Ed:
Comprehensive Sex Ed (CSE)

Are any states in the US teaching pleasure-forward sex ed? While absolutely zero states are required to address sexual pleasure, three states are at least heading in the right direction. California, Washington, and Oregon mandate "comprehensive" sex education, or CSE. What is that? CSE refers to sex ed that considers the "cognitive, emotional, physical and social aspects of sexuality."[7] Compared with abstinence-only sex ed, CSE leads to fewer pregnancies, less disease, less sexual abuse. It is scientifically accurate, is adapted to age and culture, is nondiscriminatory, and teaches *gender equality in sex*. Yes!

I have seen the transformative power of teaching CSE in countries all over the world. Girls in Kenya who better understand consent than girls in Kansas. Girls in Denmark who understand sexual pleasure is not just a boy thing—and understand it far better than girls in Delaware. Girls in Morocco who understand the importance of contraception in allowing them to stay in school better than girls in Maryland.

Arguably the three most progressive states in the United States are on board with this type of program. What is the rest of the country doing? Not much, sadly, as stats from the Guttmacher Institute on the sorry state of sex education show:[8]

- Only eighteen states require that the information in sex ed be medically accurate.
- Only ten states require that the sex ed being taught is appropriate for a student's cultural background.
- Thirty-five states allow parents to remove their child from sex education.
- Nineteen states require instruction on the importance of engaging in sexual activity only within marriage.

- Forty-six states allow the promotion of religion as part of sex education.
- Regarding teaching abstinence in sex ed:
  - 76 percent of US teens are taught abstinence as a way to prevent pregnancy and STIs.
  - Thirty-nine states and the District of Columbia require that information be provided on abstinence.
  - Ten states and Washington, DC, require that abstinence be covered in the curriculum.
  - Twenty-nine states require that abstinence be stressed!

The widespread teaching of abstinence as a viable option for birth control is not just a ridiculous denial of the fact that humans are sexual beings, it's also wildly ineffective. We know that abstinence-teaching communities do teens harm and set them up for sexual strife and problems. Studies show that, in schools and communities where abstinence is encouraged, teens experience, paradoxically, an earlier sexual debut. Teens with this type of education are also less likely to know about and to use contraception. The states with the most abstinence-heavy sex ed curriculum also have the highest teen pregnancy rates. Abstinence-forward curriculums don't work, and ones that encourage heavy parental involvement are hardly beacons of success either. Forty states and the District of Columbia require school districts to involve parents in sex education, HIV education, or both. Twenty-five states and the nation's capital require parental notification that sex education or HIV education will be provided. Six states require parental consent for students to even participate in sex education or HIV education. And thirty-five states and DC allow parents the option to remove their child from instruction.

Progressive Sex Ed from the Netherlands

Want to envision my version of a dream sex ed course? The Duke Center for Global Reproductive Health published a great article a few years ago highlighting the inadequacy of the US sex ed curriculum and compared it with sex ed in the Netherlands.[9] The same year, *The Atlantic* shared an article on *How the Dutch Do Sex Ed* with similar findings, including that Dutch sex ed begins at age four, with lessons about relationships, touching, and intimacy.[10] Seven-year-olds learn body parts. Eight-year-olds learn gender stereotypes. Eleven-year-olds learn about reproduction, safe sex, and sexual abuse.

We Americans, with our prudish ways, might worry about this methodology—*Is this too much info too soon? Is this too young to be effective?*—but data supports the Dutch approach. Teens in the Netherlands are among the top users of the birth control pill, and nine out of ten of them used contraceptives the first time they had sex. Dutch teens also have one of the lowest teen pregnancy rates in the world and low rates of STIs, including HIV. They do not have sex at an earlier age but defer until they feel ready to have sex, and by and large, they report positive first sexual experiences. This is a gynecologist's dream team, or rather, dream teen.

Sex ed in the Netherlands is a study in how a culture can be more progressive in its approach to sex. Rather than make sex taboo, the Dutch urge young people to embrace its joys, beware its perils, and learn about mutual sexual pleasure. The Dutch sex ed curriculum, similar to CSA in three US states, is based on an approach that is already being implemented in other countries as well.

What's all this got to do with the Bedroom Gap? A lot. If we can replace fear-based teaching with pleasure-based education, if we can frame sex as a lifelong source of happiness, a way to increase intimacy with a partner, a link to overall health and longevity, and a way to get closer to yourself (self-love!), then we reduce the ignorance that contributes to the Bedroom Gap affecting couples of any age, including at midlife. If young adults learn that sex is to be a positive rather than dreaded experience for both men and women right from their sexual debut, then the Bedroom Gaps of early sexual experiences and the wider midlife ones might be minimized or never occur.

Top Takeaways for Teens

1. Have sex when you want to, not when someone else wants to have sex with you.
2. Lube is your friend; use lube early and often; lube is for any age at any stage and any type of sex.
3. Know your anatomy! And know when you or your partner can and can't get pregnant.
4. Masturbation is healthy for both sexes and helps you know your own body and what sexual pleasure looks like for you.
5. Pleasure from sex should be mutual, with every partner, every time, and need not include PIV sex.

(Re)Educating the Educators and Upending Medical Education

Getting the next generation properly informed is part of improving things, but even the younger generation will need to be able to get information *from clinicians* as well. God knows we menopausal folk certainly do! Why don't clinicians know about menopause and sexual health?

Female anatomy, menopause, and sexual health, not to mention the widespread effects of menopause on pretty much every organ in the body, have been inadequately covered in medical, dental, and nursing schools. If we are going to close the Bedroom Gaps of today and prevent them from happening for tomorrow's perimenopausal women, we must get the current and future clinical communities up to speed.

The film actor Halle Berry found out the hard way just how little she (and her gynecologist!) knew about how menopause affects the female genitals. She went to the doctor with vaginal dryness (a common symptom of menopause) and was misdiagnosed with herpes. Whoa! Somebody must have skipped menopause class in medical school and again in residency. Stunned by her (mis)diagnosis, she sought another opinion and finally got some answers on just how much her body was changing now that she was in her fifties. Also, she got pissed and started advocating for more menopause awareness, in both the public and the medical spheres. Halle and I definitely agree on this: We need a sex ed overhaul for clinicians and their educators!

My patients often come to me after running into brick walls in other doctors' offices. "Part of the reason I don't know what I don't know about menopause and my sexual health is that my doctors don't ask me about it, and they don't have answers when I ask them about it," Janice tells me. "I grew up in a family where sex was never, ever discussed, and neither was aging," she shares.

Doctors are thought of as a resource for health information. But who do you go to when your doctor is in the dark? Women come to doctors for information, education, diagnosis, treatment, guidance, and referral. They wait on hold to make the appointment and then often wait weeks or months for said appointment. When the time comes, they take time off work to come to an appointment and then they wait in waiting rooms and wait again on an exam table. All for fifteen minutes with an often exhausted, time-pressed professional who was not trained in the issue they are there to discuss.

These women are sometimes listened to, and occasionally their problems are addressed and their symptoms improve; often they are dismissed, their complaints minimized or questioned, and they leave without answers, information on where to get them, or even merely feeling heard. A 2015 study from Yale found that 75 percent of women who see a doctor for help with menopause leave without treatment or answers.[11] Can you imagine if 75 percent of patients with tooth pain left the dentist without a diagnosis or treatment?

Sexual symptoms, which are even harder for many women to bring up, are too often brushed aside and women are told to "relax," or "drink some wine," or that this is just a normal part of aging. A female sexual withering with age is the party line in a medical education system that treats menopause and loss of female sexual health as an incurable event, an inevitable phase of life, a sad nod. Erectile dysfunction increases with age, but no doctor would suggest a man skip Viagra just because ED is a normal part of aging. The double standard is stunning.

Why Does the Medical Community Not Seem to Care About Menopause?

There are plenty of reasons the adoption of education in menopause and sexual health might be sluggish.

- The lack of funding to study diseases that affect women
- The exclusion of women from clinical research from 1977 until 1993
- The dramatic drop in HT use by postmenopausal women from 1999 to 2020, largely driven by the WHO study findings described earlier in this book

- The lack of acknowledgment by medical institutions that menopause and sexual health are important to overall human health

Lack of Funding

Despite women representing over half the population, research that benefits women has historically been underfunded. Only about 8.8 percent of the NIH research spending was directed toward women's health from 2013 to 2023. In December 2024, the National Academies of Sciences Engineering and Medicine (NASEM) released a congressionally mandated report assessing the state of women's health research. The report showed an urgent need to increase funding for women's health, establish a new women's health institute within the NIH, and increase the grants and research that could lead to breakthrough science in women's health.[12]

Lack of Women in Clinical Trials

Most clinical research focuses on men of European ancestry. This has downstream implications galore—treatments, medication dosages, even what doctors learn from medical school textbooks are all based on white men. By excluding women from participating in research, and by not specifically analyzing data through a gender lens, we miss opportunities to learn about how a given medication or treatment might work differently in women.

How did we get here? In 1977, in the wake of the thalidomide disaster, the FDA advised against including women of childbearing age in clinical trials to avoid potential harm to the fetus of a trial participant. The impact of this lengthy exclusion of women from medical trials limited our understanding of how disease processes and treatments differed for women, especially since there are:

- Diseases and conditions that *only* affect women (endometriosis, uterine fibroids)
- Diseases and conditions that *more commonly* affect women (Alzheimer's, stroke, osteoporosis, depression, urinary tract infections, and thyroid disease)
- Diseases and conditions that affect women and men *differently* (heart disease and stroke)

In 1993 the NIH reversed the 1977 policy and required the inclusion of women and ethnic and racial minorities in clinical research studies. Hooray! Except that although many of these studies now included female subjects, they *failed to evaluate the sex-based differences in the data*, making the inclusion of women little more than checking the diversity box. In 2016 the NIH mandated the consideration of sex as a biological variable. While NIH-funded trials showed increasing female participation from 2013–2018, there was no increase at all in the sex-based analysis within those studies.[13] Aaaaaargh!!! What good is it to include women in a study if you don't use the sex differences as one lens through which to look at the data?

When HRT Left Town

When the Women's Health Initiative was formed, it was in the spirit of looking at disease states that affected women, including heart disease and breast cancer. But when the WHI trial data was published in 2002, indicating concerns about harmful effects (did someone say cancer?!) of hormone replacement therapy (HT), the world took notice, and hormone use for treatment of menopausal symptoms vanished overnight. Even though these findings have been largely disproven due to flawed study methods, HT use by postmenopausal women dropped dramatically from 26.9 percent to 4.7 percent between 1999 and 2020 and has really never recovered.[14] What cruel irony that an NIH initiative aimed to improve understanding of women's health backfired in such a detrimental way. The loss of health benefits from twenty years of women not using HT is hard to quantify but is massive to say the least. One study estimated that over a ten-year span, approximately fifty thousand postmenopausal women died prematurely by avoiding estrogen therapy after a hysterectomy.[15] Read that stunning statistic again. And this represents just a fraction of the actual toll of disease burden, hospitalizations, and deaths since 2002 because of the drop in HT use. How many heart attacks, hip fractures, and UTIs could have been prevented had the WHI not sounded the false alarm about HT?

It's Just Aging, Deal with It

In the wake of the uproar over hormone replacement therapy and with HT prescriptions a thing of the past, medical education and practicing clinicians basically reverted to the idea that menopause is a natural state and that women should just accept the consequences. This was a convenient solution—what's easier, after all, than entirely ignoring a huge medical blind spot?—and explains the lack of teaching of menopause and its consequences, including sexual consequences, in medical education. It also explains the dismissive attitude that persists even today among many practicing clinicians.

You can see why any effort to change medical education in a meaningful and efficient way for women's health, especially sexual issues of older women, will be an uphill climb. Enter Doctor Wen Shen. Although not (yet!) a household name, Shen is quietly moving the needle forward at the level of medical education. Wen Shen was a mentor during my own residency in Baltimore and now directs the Women's Wellness & Healthy Aging Program at Johns Hopkins Hospital.

Recently, I asked her to answer a simple question because I was badly hoping to hear a wise, reassuring answer from someone in the thick of medical education.

What would you do to overhaul the medical education system so that medically trained clinicians would be better educated about and more willing to discuss, diagnose, and treat menopause issues and issues relating to female sexual health?

Wen Shen's answer was as sharp as I expected it to be: "Maria, women will never be able to get help for sexual issues related to menopause until we get *menopause* itself into the educational curriculum of medical students," she says.

If she were in charge, what would she do? "I would designate one or two lectures solely on menopause and make it mandatory in the curricula of all medical school, physician assistant, and nurse practitioner programs; the learning objectives would have to include how menopause impacts the whole body, the physical and mental health of women, so that this would plant the seeds in the brains of the students that menopause can have far-reaching effects."

Shen goes on, "I would mandate that there be menopause education in all residency programs, in every specialty and subspecialty, because we literally have estrogen receptors everywhere in our body. But I would start with good, deep, hands-on experiences for ob/gyn residents, internal medicine and family medicine residents. Get that in place, then dream of spreading that education outward into all specialties."

Shen paused, thought a bit, then added, "The way this is taught is important. I would not want dry lectures; I would want residents to rotate through a real menopause clinic so they could see how much and in how many ways menopause patients suffer. I want residents to hear the patients say 'something is really wrong with me, I think I am going crazy. I miss work because my hot flashes are relentless. I used to love sex and now I dread it. My husband left me because we stopped having sex.' Then I want the residents to see the same women come back with the massive improvements that can be attained with treatments like hormone therapy. I would want them to see the various manifestations of menopause, from palpitations, joint pains, burning mouth, formication, hair loss, dry eyes to pain and bleeding with intercourse to loss of libido, so they could understand that whatever their future specialty, they will likely encounter patients whose symptoms relate to menopause.[16] The problem is that today there are simply not enough menopause clinics in the US, so even well-intentioned residency programs might not have access to a menopause clinic."[17]

I'll add my own gripe to hers here—there are simply not enough *clinicians* trained to staff the not enough menopause clinics. I asked Dr. Shen about her oft-quoted survey from 2012 that contained stunning statistics about the state of affairs of medical education with respect to menopause and wondered whether those statistics have changed or improved since 2012. Shen was clear: "There have been two similar surveys since mine in 2012, and the statistics have barely changed; we have had almost *no improvement* in the medical education systems with respect to menopause and sexual health, so sadly the stats from my survey in 2012 are still applicable."[18]

Some of the sobering stats from Dr. Shen's survey on menopause education include:

- Only 20 percent of residency programs had a menopause curriculum
- Only 16 percent of residency programs had a menopause clinic
- 66–79 percent of residents said they needed more learning on the nuts and bolts of menopause

And Dr. Shen's personal favorite:

- 90 percent of fourth year residents, doctors who were about to graduate and go out into the world to practice, said they did not feel comfortable discussing or treating menopause. *Ninety percent.*

Dr. Stephanie Faubion is another widely respected menopause expert; her 2019 study looked at gaps in menopause education and found that 20 percent of ob/gyn, internal medicine, and family practice residents had *no education in menopause*; that *less than 7 percent* of those residents felt adequately prepared to manage menopausal issues; and that around two-thirds of the residents gave the wrong answer to a basic question about menopause treatment.[19] Come on, doctors. We can do better than this! No wonder women are flocking to the internet or social media for information and buying (sometimes dubious) treatments online. The menopause market is exploding, projected to reach between $24 and $600 billion by 2030, and at least some of that retail bonanza is driven by what doctors *aren't* doing or hearing or treating in the exam room.[20]

This is totally unacceptable, right? Since 2012 humanity has seen the widespread adoption of smartphones, reusable rockets for space travel, advances in self-driving cars, breakthroughs in stem cell research, CRISPR gene editing technology, and the development of artificial intelligence (AI); Amazon has revolutionized e-commerce, and Uber has transformed transportation. But we can't make changes so that future health care providers know what happens to 100 percent of women as they age? Pathetic.

Dr. Shen makes another sobering point: "Women with menopausal symptoms have historically been relegated to psychiatric care—the hysterical woman, the woman with neuroses." This is convenient. It spares the clinician from having to learn—or even just guess—whether their patients' symptoms have a hormonal basis, and it saves them from having to be responsible for knowing the hormonal basis for treatment. Remember the unfortunate 1995 patient of mine from an earlier chapter who I referred to a psychiatrist? Even I suffered from this lack of training, and so did my patients.

Doctors and Sex Talk

Why else don't clinicians talk about menopause, and especially about sex and menopause? When asked why, some clinicians say they are very uncomfortable talking about sex in general. They bring the tenets of their own upbringing—"we never mentioned it at home; we were taught not to talk about it, that sex is a dirty and shameful subject"—into their dealings with patients. This underscores the need for societal change at the earliest levels (comprehensive sex ed!). We need to remove the stigma and shame surrounding sex and allow health classes and medical school educations and families to be able to discuss sex honestly.

Physicians also cite that they don't discuss sexual issues with patients due to lack of time in a busy schedule, which suggests to me that sexual health has not been prioritized as part of physical and mental health. Unlike readers of this book, residents haven't learned (and so don't adopt this in their clinical repertoire) that an active sex life has been associated with reduced heart disease, less depression, increased happiness, and longer lifespan.[21]

The result of poor education in menopause and sexual health: Too many women are essentially forced to compete in a twisted version of a menopausal medical decathlon: The perimenopausal or postmenopausal woman might have to go see the cardiologist for palpitations, the rheumatologist for joint stiffness, the internist for fatigue, and the psychiatrist for her anxiety and moodiness, and so on and so on. Many, if not all these specialists, often fail to consider that the little almond-sized ovaries in her pelvis are unleashing the hormonal chaos or hormonal absence that is causing many of these health and quality of life issues, many of which can be improved with a single prescription for HT. With such a massive knowledge gap, it is no wonder that many Bedroom Gap problems are very unlikely to be broached and even less likely to be treated by your clinician.

Sex Ed for Doctors—Better Late Than Never?

The lack of training in menopause among clinicians is a real problem. What about training specifically in sexuality? A 2016 study looked at the perceptions of US medical residents regarding the amount and usefulness of their training in sexuality, which turned out to be inadequate in both content and amount. The residents reported that their training was usually under ten *hours* out of four to five *years* of training—a wink and a nod at best. And 60 percent received minimal to no educational training *at all* in sexual issues.[22]

And much like inadequate high school sex ed we discussed earlier in this chapter, the content for residents was also focused mostly on STIs, HIV, anatomy, and physiology. There was no time given for meaningful education about consent, LGBTQ+ populations, desire, pleasure, orgasm. No training about sex in cancer survivors or transgender patients, never mind any attention paid to understanding what is happening in the bedroom due to social media and online dating trends. This is woefully inadequate.

It's no wonder present-day clinicians are reluctant to address sexual issues. They simply aren't prepared to discuss what they *haven't* been taught. Pediatricians get training in puberty issues so that they can talk with teens about how the body changes at the beginning of our reproductive years; we should do the same for the clinicians who are caring for women at the close of their reproductive capacity.

How Can Doctors Be Better at Helping Us with Sexual Issues?

1. Be better listeners.
2. Be empathic: Give permission to share intimate issues with body and facial cues.
3. Be informed: Learn and train through the International Society for the Study of Women's Sexual Health (ISSWSH) and the World Association of Sexual Health (WAS).
4. Know where to refer patients for sexual counseling and therapy: Find trained professionals at the American Association of Sexuality Educators, Counselors, and Therapists (AASECT).

We need to start with physicians' behavior in the exam room. One study showed that, on average, physicians interrupt the patient after just eighteen seconds; in another study, it was only eleven seconds.[23] While most interruptions are cooperative, meaning they contribute to the outcome of the conversation, they are also more likely to be made by men interrupting women.[24] The issue is complex because there are gender roles (are men more comfortable interrupting women?) and societal hierarchy (is a doctor always at the top of the food chain in a one-on-one interaction?) at play here as well as the undeniable reality that even the best-intentioned clinicians are trying to conduct a meaningful visit in an often impossibly short time frame.

Moreover, sexual health training for clinicians needs to encompass a myriad of issues and topics; we need to move past covering only sex for white heterosexual, monogamous couples. We doctors need to embrace today's sexual diversity, including subjects like nonbinary gender identification, transgender sexual issues (especially after gender reassignment surgery), polyamorous relationships, online dating, sexual issues faced by cancer survivors, and changes in current sexual preferences.

We have already discussed the disturbing increased heterosexual male interest in both choking and anal sex, which is reflective of more recent shifts in pornography scripting. If your recent Tinder date wanted to have anal sex or get a bit rough, would you be comfortable asking your doctor about this? Would your doctor be capable, never mind comfortable, having this kind of sex talk with you? Too few clinicians have had the kind of training that prepares them for their patients' real life sexual issues. Too few can speak with you about sex after mastectomy, or organ transplant, or how to have responsible sex with an HIV or hepatitis diagnosis. Too few can discuss and recommend specific toys for self-love to a widowed patient, discuss polyamory STI testing regimens, the right lube for anal sex, or dilators that might help a transwoman with a neovagina.

Apologies to you all on behalf of all us clinicians. To find a clinician who really does know and care about female sexual health, check out ISSWSH. Remember Irwin Goldstein, the entrepreneurial urologist who helped Pfizer change our views on ED and brand Viagra into a blockbuster? Well, he is still around, and he actually has been a leader in the movement to improve female sexual health. He is a major figure at ISSWSH, and his center in San Diego is the go-to place for women with complex sexual disorders of desire, arousal, pain, and lack of orgasm.

Advocates for better education and better understanding are out there—advocates like Doctors Shen and Goldstein and so many others. And we've spent the last several chapters training ourselves to be our own advocates. Pretty soon, there will be an army of us. If we make enough noise, demanding to be heard, to be listened to, to be seen, then the medical institutions and the education systems will have to listen to us.

There is some good news—there are already changes happening on the consumer side of things. Why? Because, it turns out that forty-five-to-sixty-year-old women have quite a lot of spending power and the demand for women's health everything is through the roof. The Femtech Market was valued in 2023 at around $50 billion and is expected to grow to $135 billion by 2032.[25] And as we all know, when there's money to be made, the private sector is very good at paying attention.

Chapter 9

❧

Toys, Lube, Erotica, and Virtual Reality

We have built a strong case for the changes that need to be made in the public sector to improve sexual education, at all ages and in all places, to help close the Bedroom Gap.

We've talked desire, pleasure, porn, and orgasm. You should be feeling pretty prepped and pumped to tackle whatever Bedroom Gap you might be struggling with. But in case you need more of a nudge, let's give you even more tools to work with.

We'll start with some "homework" to get the sexy part of your brain engaged: erotic literature, audio and visual porn, steamy podcasts. Then we'll look at in-the-bedroom helpers: sex toys and lubes. Finally, we'll go next level with a look at the Sextech boom and how we can use artificial intelligence and even virtual reality for augmented and remote sexual experiences that work with our lives and needs today. But first, a look (way) back at the human need to be aroused by visual images and the written word.

Erotica in Art

When asked about the difference between art and eroticism, Pablo Picasso answered, "But—there is no difference.... Art is never chaste; one should keep it away from all innocent ignoramuses. People insufficiently prepared for art should never be allowed close to art. Yes, art is dangerous. If it is chaste, it is not art."[1]

Sexual interest piqued by visual images is hardly new. Erotica has been a part of the human experience since the beginning of recorded time. The ancient Greeks and Romans created public frescoes and sculptures depicting homosexuality, fellatio, cunnilingus, even threesomes. The Kama Sutra, published in India in the second century AD, is a classic Hindu Sanskrit book that describes many aspects of love, sexuality, and emotional fulfillment. It contains instructions for how to be a good wife, tips on personal grooming, and cures for sexual problems such as how to cultivate sensual pleasure and sexual desire. It also describes sixty-four sex acts, including many different sexual positions, which is what it is most known for in the Western world.

From 100 to 800 AD, the Moche people of Peru created amazing pre-Columbian pottery that you can still see at the Museo Larco in Lima. It depicts penises and vaginas as water pitchers pouring forth what might represent sexual fluids. They depict gay male anal intercourse, lesbian sex, heterosexual couples, and threesomes. I remember visiting this exhibit, and a museum guard scolding me and shooing me toward another room when I looked a bit too long at one well-endowed water pitcher. Maybe he thought the art was inappropriate for a young woman or felt uncomfortable watching me admiring the phallus-shaped clay jug. Maybe he had pottery penis envy!

Shunga, a type of Japanese erotic art, existed in the Edo period in Japan (1603–1867) in the form of woodblock prints or handmade scrolls. Spectacularly rendered, shunga art was owned by both men and women, since couples were often separated for long periods of time due to jobs and wartime circumstances.[2] I love the progressive thinking that the women would need erotic imagery as well.

We can find erotica in art almost as far back as we can find art itself, but of course the art form has evolved over the years. While sex-themed pottery and prints served as daily reminders of the erotic side of life for centuries, in the eighteenth century, English readers were treated to a more thorough and descriptive erotic experience. 1748 saw the publication of the first full-length pornographic novel in the English language. *Memoirs of a Woman of Pleasure*, otherwise known as *Fanny Hill*, tells the story of a girl who arrives from the countryside to Georgian London and becomes a prostitute. I first read *Fanny Hill* as a literature student living in Paris in my twenties. Neither stuffy nor outdated, *Fanny Hill* looks at the meaning of sensuality; it is an enduring work of erotic literature and a great read at any age. Despite the author, John Cleland, never mentioning Fanny's genitals by name, there are plenteous references to parts swelling and blooming and blood rushing. The book, which covers voyeuristic sex, masochism, and bisexuality among other things, was denounced by the bishop of London who, ironically, was a frequent patron of the same bawdy establishments it described.

Another British erotica bestseller was anonymously published in 1888. *My Secret Life* is a memoir of the sexual experiences of a gentleman in Victorian London over the span of forty years. The massive work, four thousand pages long and over one million words in eleven volumes, recites the many sexual liaisons of "Walter," a self-described sex addict. In the memoir, we learn about the social classes of the times and about London's houses of prostitution, and of course about sex with everyone from servants to working-class women to individuals belonging to London's upper crust. No way was I reading *that* monster tome in my twenties—there were real live Parisian men (and women) to get to know!

In nineteenth-century France, meanwhile, erotic images were being recorded as daguerreotypes, the predecessors of modern photographs. The earliest known example was produced in 1846, of a man inserting his penis into a woman's vagina.

The silent film era began around 1894, and by 1896 the first pornographic film had been made, depicting sexual intercourse. The oldest surviving hardcore porn film is a French production titled *À L'Ecu d'Or ou la Bonne Auberge* (1908), in which a woman pleasures herself with a dildo, then is joined by another woman and a man with whom she has a threesome, complete with oral sex and intercourse. Leave it to the French to be cinematically sexually progressive! The history of erotic art could comprise another hundred pages of this book. Suffice to say, eroticism has been the subject of human artistic expression for millennia and continues today.

Erotica Today . . . Is Porn All We've Got?

The "artistic" expression of sex today, for most of us, unfortunately mostly means porn. One third of all internet traffic, at certain times of the day, is porn. And the modern pornography industry is controlled by a handful of (male founded, male run, male owned, just saying) for-profit companies whose goal is neither ethical nor accurate representation of real-world sex. It certainly is not about sex from a female perspective. Porn today is loud, aggressive, and in your face. It is coercive, physical, more violent with trends such as ATM (ass-to-mouth), gagging (a penis thrust so far down a woman's throat she gags), and (usually female-received) choking. In one study, the two most common names women were called in porn scenes were "bitch" and "slut"; worse even than the name-calling was the women's reactions to the slurs in the sex scenes—their scripted response was either neutral or positive.[3]

As we learned in the last chapter, because the sex ed we are offering to our children is so inadequate, or in some cases is altogether absent, kids are learning about sex from porn. Period. Those kids, in too few years, will become sexually active teens and adults. Is it any wonder, then, that Bedroom Gaps—gendered differences in sexual expectations—develop even when we are just beginning to have sex, and widen/worsen when our bodies change with age?

How do *you* feel when you look at or listen to erotic expressions today? If porn is our version of erotic art, is it doing its job? Is it titillating you, getting you excited about sex? Or does it concern you? Does it represent a perpetuation of patriarchal control and the degradation of females?

It is understandable to feel squeamish, repulsed, embarrassed when you look at or listen to pornography today. How can you find erotic expression that pleases you in a world where vile, degrading pornography is pervasive and just a click away? Where the sexual exploitation of children and unsafe sexual practices have been filmed for profit, and where it seems every click on Pornhub is more degrading to women than the last?

Female-Forward Porn

Enter Erica Lust, an award-winning filmmaker and author whose sex-positive, intimacy-allowing, female-forward films have challenged (but unfortunately not changed) the status quo in adult entertainment. Her films include, in her own words, "relatable characters, beautiful cinematography, diverse and empowering narratives on porn, sexuality and pleasure."[4] Lust describes the male-created, male dominated porn industry, which she calls "Big Porn," as ethically bereft, and all about "concentrating power and maximizing profit." Lust blames Big Porn for the "bad education" that begets inaccurate portrayals of sex, which in turn begets the misaligned sexual expectations and unfulfilled fantasies of adults. In short, Big Porn—our society's mass consumed, most prevalent source of sexual information—perpetuates the centuries old patriarchal sexual scripts that massively contribute to the Bedroom Gap. But there are, of late, some alternatives, thank goodness!

Sex in Words
If you aren't comfortable diving into the world of pornographic cinema, even films made with women in mind, perhaps you can get your toes wet with the medium most women find palatable: the written word. It has long been known that men's brains are turned on by visual pornographic images, whereas women seem to prefer a more private experience, one where they can lean into fantasy and their imagination. Enter the romance novel.[5] There really is something for everyone's erotic taste: from the hot young teacher having sex with his student's mom to the vampire getting down and fangy with her besotted victims, there is fantasy-filled lit erotica to suit any taste. Search "erotic literature," then add a descriptor such as vampire or hot teacher or horseback ride and see what comes up. You can also search "best women's erotica of the year."

AudioPorn: Aural Sex Goes Mainstream
A natural development of erotic literature in this era of the internet is audio porn. Audio porn—sites and apps with erotic stories, and erotic podcasts—leverages the potential of the spoken word to excite women. Despite the somewhat off-putting name, audio porn is simply erotic literature read to you, and it is a wonderfully private and relaxing, or arousing, way to consume erotic content at your own pace

and in the privacy of your own headspace. I love recommending it to my patients because all you need is a smartphone or computer and ideally a set of headphones. Bathtub, candles, vibrator are optional!

Now that you're armed with loads of female-forward sexual content, it's likely that sex will be on your brain, in a great way. But bringing your best self to the bedroom involves knowing yourself sexually and knowing what feels good. Self-pleasure, sex toys, and lube are all ways to up your game. You may masturbate regularly, with or without toys; you may never ever have done so. Either way, read on to give the midlife sex you're having a little tune up. Let's start with masturbation, then move on to toys or, as some folks call them, sex tools.

Masturbation

Really the best way to improve your relationship to sex is to get to know yourself, sexually. Self-pleasure can begin with something as simple as looking closely at your naked body and touching whatever part feels good to be touched. The more you touch your own body, the clearer it will be as to what feels good to you, and what doesn't. If it feels too awkward, start with G-rated masturbation (remember from the Five *M*'s?), meaning touch a body part that isn't genital or erogenous, like the inner part of your arm.

Just stroke the inner aspect of your arm and appreciate not just how it relaxes you but also maybe how it makes you feel tingly and good. Maybe graduate to applying vibration to the same area with one of the toys we'll talk about in a minute. You can eventually graduate from arm to breast, and from breast to vulva, or just stick with whatever feels good to you. This sounds basic, but it is exactly what you need to know to be able to teach a sex partner what you like.

One of my favorite resources is OMGYes, a website that gathers data from interviewing thousands of women about sexual habits and what they do and what they like. From all that information, they have created tutorials and videos to help with many aspects of sexual experience, including masturbation. The site also addresses sexual communication, variations of clitoral touching, anal touch, pleasure from showers and baths, how best to use toys, penetration techniques, and other topics that make you realize other women like many of the same things you do! There is a one-time fee to access all the knowledge and community of OMGYes. I highly suggest you check it out.

Great Sex Toys

How do I introduce a sex toy into my relationship? What if my partner feels threatened or uncomfortable with this? Where do I even buy one? What if my kids see this? I get asked these questions all the time. Until we destigmatize sex and pleasure, we can't be comfortable with toys, lube, bondage, or porn. Lest we've forgotten, sex is how we all got here! Remind your partner that you love your sex life with him/her/them but that you also love the idea of *trying new things together.* Perhaps share that you have a desire to have "blended" orgasms—sensations felt intensely both inside and outside the body. You can either (1) present a toy you purchased to your partner or (2) ask to go shopping for the toy together.

Sex toys can be grouped into types:

1. **G-spot vibrators, or wand vibrators:** These are usually shaped like a penis, inserted into the vagina, or slightly curved, like the Njoy Pure Wand, or Lelo's Gigi 2.
2. **Clitoral stimulators:** These offer many different ways to focus excitement at the clitoris, from vibration, motion,

and sound waves to suction (Dame Aer, Lelo Dot, Lelo Sona 2).

3. **Rabbit vibrators:** With two vibrating bunny "ears," these offer simultaneous internal and external stimulation (Lovehoney Happy Rabbit, Babeland Lioness, Lelo Soraya 2, and Cosara Triple Vibe).

4. **Starter Toys:** Some toys are meant for general stimulation and can be used anywhere on the body—I love these as a place to start if you are new to self-pleasure. They are never shaped like a penis, are nonthreatening to use, and feel good even just to place on your tummy for relaxation or on your breasts or inner thighs for low-level feel good. (Pom by Dame, Vibe by Maude, Mimi by Je Joue, and Iroha+ line by Tenga are all high end, aesthetically pleasing, beautifully designed vibrators that don't look like sex toys at all. You could leave them on your dresser or bathroom counter and not feel embarrassed. Vesper by Crave is actually worn as a necklace, looks like a golf tee, and is USB charged.)

5. **Air Toys:** These use air to generate pulses and are often very quiet. Examples include Satisfyer Pro, Womanizer Premium (uses air instead of sonic pulses), and Sona Cruise 2. Lelo's Sona Cruise 2 merits a shout-out for its "intuitive, responsive" function. This clitoral stimulator has "cruise control," that is, when the device is pressed harder against the body, it releases extra power as "sonic pulses which resonate deep into the internal structure of the clitoris."[6]

6. **Couples' Vibrators:** Models such as Eva2 by Dame can be worn and provide vibrations to both partners at once.

7. **Cock Rings/Anal Play** (Phanxy and WeVibe cock rings, Silent Fun anal vibrator, Dibe vibrator/prostate massager, with a heat function): These sound intimidating, but maybe you can work your way up to this after you and your partner have explored the previous options.
8. **Fingertip Vibrator** (Fin by Dame): Minimalist but great easy fun.

Other nice options to spice things up include body oils and massage oils. The high-end sexual wellness company Maude makes a soy massage candle—as it burns, the wax becomes a massage oil. I love this idea! Companies like Astraèa and Foria make body oils that can be used as massage oils or personal lubricants (more on this in a moment) that include CBD, which they claim can be helpful with relaxation, good for the skin, and orgasm enhancing!

Wedge pillows, used to elevate hips during sex, can be fun or just plain helpful, especially if mobility is an issue after surgery or from arthritis; two nice ones are sold by Maude in washable linen and Dame with a washable cover.

Arousal serums usually contain ingredients that cause blood vessels to dilate, which facilitates swelling of tissue and gives a warm feeling; other ingredients can provide a bit of tingle to sensitive areas. Compounding pharmacies make versions called O Cream or Scream Cream, and there are over-the-counter versions in abundance.

Edible libido-enhancing gummies and supplements are all over the internet; for men, the most effective ones contain L-Arginine and Maca. For women the supplements or gummies should contain L-Arginine, Fenugreek extract, and Ginkgo Biloba. I will warn you that most commercial supplements on the market fail tests of purity or effectiveness, so buyer beware.

The Lowdown on Lube

Lube is nothing to be ashamed of. Using lube does not mean you are "all dried up, past your prime, or just not turned on," as my patients ashamedly tell me, looking at the ground with a defeated posture. Don't fall for that crap—lube is your friend! Wetter is better at any age, so lube should be part of sex at every age. If you are dreading bringing lube into your sex life because, again, your partner might take offense or feel inadequate or question your interest, you can put a positive spin on it this way: "I loved our sex the other day and was thinking this aloe vera lube might make it even more fun. Let's try it and see. If you don't like it, we can try something else, but I think it would make things even better." Show a lube you choose to your partner or go internet "shopping" together and look forward to your lube delivery as an excuse to try it out. Don't hide it away and sheepishly sneak it under the covers in shame. This is your body, right now, and your bringing lube to bed is a statement not of failure but of embracing your desire to have comfortable sex and your right to pleasurable sex. Keep it on your nightstand as a proud statement to your partner that you welcome the chance to use it. There's always the nightstand drawer when you need it for privacy!

Lube 101: Three Lube Lessons
Lube Lesson 1: Different types of lubes have pros and cons. Here is a quick lowdown:

1. **Water-based:** The most common type of lube, and the most "natural feeling," water-based lubes come with or without glycerin. Glycerin can give a slightly sweet taste to the lube, which some people prefer, but if you are prone to yeast infections, you might want to avoid lubes

that contain it. Water-based lube is thin in consistency and so does not last long; you may need to reapply it or blend it with a silicone-based lube so it lasts longer. It's safe to use with condoms and sex toys made of silicone.

2. **Silicone-based:** These lubes are a great option if you want some sexual fun in the shower or any play in the water; it lasts longer but feels less natural. Great for people with skin sensitivities since it is hypoallergenic; it has a slippery, silky feel and a thicker consistency than water-based lubes. Uberlube is one of my favorite silicone lube options, and it can be used to prevent chafing during fitness workouts or even as a glossy hair gel—no kidding!

3. **Oil-based:** These lubes are even thicker than either water or silicone-based lubes, and they stay put, but they can promote yeast infections in some women, and they can degrade condoms.

4. **Natural alternatives:**
    a. **Edible oils:** Coconut oil is the most common, but you can also use other edible oils such as grapeseed, avocado, or olive oil; just remember they can damage condoms, as well as stain sheets and clothing.
    b. **Aloe vera:** One of my favorite lubes to recommend is Aloe Cadabra—it is a fan favorite among my Patient Posse, as is Good Clean Love Almost Naked.

Lube Lesson 2: The type of condom you use dictates the lube choice.

1. **Latex condoms:** Only use water or silicone-based lubes; avoid oil-based lubes, which can degrade the condom and lead to an oops!

2. **Polyisoprene (PI) condoms:** Ditto. Polyisoprene is a synthetic rubber, like latex, and can break down with the use of oil-based lubricants. SKYN condoms are a popular brand made from PI and are great for people with latex allergies.

3. **Polyurethane condoms:** These can be broken down by silicone (go figure) so only water- or oil-based lubes should be used with these; examples include Trojan Non-Latex Bareskin and Skyn Original, a polyurethane and polyisoprene blend.

4. **Lambskin/Sheepskin condoms:** Any type of lube works!

5. **Sex Aids/Toys: Remember:** No silicone lube with silicone toys, except for the brand Love Not War, which has created a type of silicone that is okay to use with silicone toys.

Lube Lesson 3: Check the label!
In general, the fewer the ingredients, the healthier the lube. The World Health Organization recommends a lube with pH of 4.5 and low osmolality (less than 1200 mOsm/kg).[7] Ingredients to avoid in a lube:

- **Parabens:** Somewhat linked to cancer.
- **Nonoxynol-9:** Can cause genital irritation, sperm damage, toxic shock syndrome.
- **Benzocaine:** Used for numbing but irritates genital tissue.
- **Fragrances/flavors:** Personal choice here, but in general these are ingredients that could be irritating.
- **Glycerin:** Can promote yeast infections.
- **Chlorhexidine gluconate:** A preservative that can alter the vaginal microbiome.

- **Petrochemicals** such as petroleum, propylene glycol, and polyethylene glycol are endocrine disrupters, interfering with hormone production and are linked to inflammation.
  - ⊚ Petroleum products can promote bacterial vaginosis, an imbalance of bacteria that causes unpleasant odor.[8]
  - ⊚ Propylene glycol can be responsible for allergic skin reactions.

The bottom line is that lube can be a helpful and fun-enhancing part of your sex life, a Bedroom Gap closer, and a bridge to comfortable sex at any age, especially in midlife and beyond. Choose your lube with care and, like voting, lube early and lube often.

The Future of Sex: SexTech, Teledildonics, and VR Porn

The sexual wellness market is booming. The options for toys and lube have skyrocketed, as have the number of TEDx talks devoted to sex. Although the explosion of pornography on the internet has upsides

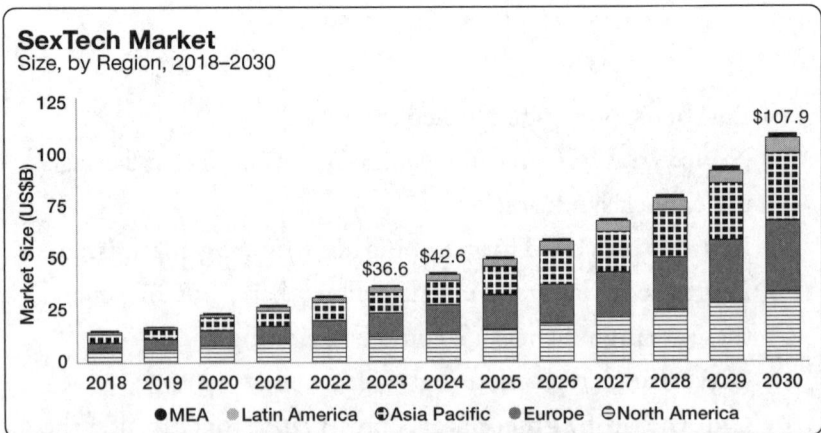

SexTech Market
Size, by Region, 2018–2030

$36.6 $42.6 $107.9

●MEA ●Latin America ◑Asia Pacific ●Europe ⊖North America

https://www.grandviewresearch.com/industry-analysis/sextech-market-report

and downsides, all this increase in the commercialization of sex has aligned nicely to stimulate the sex market (see graph).

As of 2024, the global sex tech market was estimated at $42.59 billion and is projected to reach between $100 and $122 billion by 2031.

The market growth has been a perfect storm of sorts, the result of several overlapping factors:

1. The boom in dating apps has meant more couples are getting together more easily, with more efficiency.
2. The legalization of gay marriage has led to a more visible LGBTQ community and a readiness to purchase toys and aids for their unique sexual needs.
3. Increased per capita income in developing countries has meant more disposable income for luxury purchases such as items devoted to well-being and pleasure, like sex toys.
4. Increased attention being paid to well-being and self-care for menopausal-age women includes a new focus on sexual wellness for older women.
5. The COVID pandemic led to a huge increase in sales of sex toys, which has persisted. The isolation of the pandemic inspired a need for solo sexual pleasure and accelerated awareness of "technology-enhanced intimacy solutions." Sex toy sales during this period doubled in countries like Colombia, Australia, Denmark, and the UK, and even tripled in New Zealand.[9]
6. Developments in Sextech devices that now are app-controlled and use AI and Bluetooth enhanced user experience.

The Future of Sex Toys Has Already Arrived

What exactly are these "technological advancements" in the sex toy world? Let's use a compare and contrast scenario. A vibrator from your past might have been made of hard shiny plastic, shaped like an erect penis or a rocket, had an on/off button, and was awkwardly noisy. It was often giant and off-putting in terms of size and its noisy jackhammer-like vibration.

Vibrators today are often quieter, are usually waterproof, and are aesthetically designed with medical grade silicone, which is soft to touch and easy to clean. They come equipped with variable settings and vibratory patterns. The giant straight shaft, likely designed by men as (their idea of) a woman's ultimate fantasy, has been replaced by either curved designs or designs that preferentially stimulate the G-spot and/or the clitoris. Some companies promote their toys as eco-friendly, vegan, and carbon-neutral in their manufacturing processes.

Technological Advancements in Sex Toys

1. Customization: Newer toys have dynamic responses (meaning that the sensation changes depending on how you use the toy) and use AI for personalization—the device "learns" what you like and sets that as preferential settings.
2. User experience: Older toys provided basic sensations requiring manual adjustment; newer toys "learn" the user's preferences and patterns of use and adapt.
3. Interactivity: AI now syncs toys to videos and interactive games and is also used in remote app-based controls.
4. Long-distance control: This allows a partner to control sex play with a sex toy via an app that is used long-distance.

The recent increased interest in and acceptance of sex toys and the launch of several new, well-funded relevant companies has made it easier and more acceptable for women to embrace sexual wellness as a part of total health and well-being. What is out there for women wanting to elevate their sex game?

From Smartphones to Smart Dildos

Samantha and Jason were totally into each other sexually; both divorced, both in their late forties, they met on a dating app and were really excited about their relationship. There was just one problem: Sam lives in San Diego and Jason in Boston, and we all know that long distance can be quite a buzzkill for sex. Enter Lovense, a company that makes smartphone-connected sex toys that allow you to pleasure your partner remotely, even *very* remotely.

How exactly does that work? Lovense sells sex toys that can be used alone or in person with a partner and are controlled by an app. Great, cool. Now at least you can use that smartphone you can't seem to get out of the bedroom for some sexual fun!

But Lovense also has a Lovense Remote app, and this is something quite different. It allows you to use the app to control your partner's sex toy and, in turn, their sexual experience, remotely. You can also link your partner's sex toy to your sex toy, so that the way you use your sex toy will affect your partner's sex toy. Let me give you an example. If Sam in San Diego uses her vibrator with quick thrusts into her vagina, the masturbatory vibrations and squeezing of her partner's sex toy in Boston will increase in intensity; if in turn her partner Jason increases the speed of thrusting with his sex toy while in Boston, Samantha's dildo in San Diego will vibrate more intensely.

How exactly would a long-distance session work? First, you pair each toy with an internet-connected device using the Lovense

Remote app. Message or call your partner either through any video chat service, or through Lovense's proprietary software. Start video chatting and begin to use the toys when you are ready. The toys will respond to your movements and send the feedback to your partner's toy. There is a learning curve, no doubt, so keep your sense of humor and your expectations moderate when you get started.

When I first learned about some of these options, I presumed cost would be a barrier to utilizing these dueling teledildonics.[10] Sold together, MAX 2 and Nora cost $179. Not cheap, but cheaper than a plane ticket!

Next Level Play:
Teledildonics plus VR Porn

No need to stop there. This type of high-tech sex play can get even more, well, tech-y. Teledildonics—virtual sex encounters using networked electronic sex toys to mimic and extend human sexual interaction, like the one I just described—can be used in conjunction with virtual reality porn (VR porn). Very few users of teledildonics use them in conjunction with adult VR content, mostly due to cost, but also because few people have knowledge about this new niche within the porn industry. The effectiveness of VR porn, in terms of feeling like you are "really there" with the porn actors, and in terms of the level of sexual arousal that develops, has been studied for both men and women. For both sexes, sexual presence and sexual arousal were significantly higher from watching VR videos than regular 2D videos.[11] Game on!

Virtual reality is a simulated experience that uses pose tracking to create an immersive video experience.[12] Users wear three-dimensional "goggles" called near-eye displays and can use these to watch videos, including porn. The appeal is obvious: Watching porn is usually a private experience, and goggles that put you right in the middle of the "action" is a more private and personal experience compared with watching erotic content on your laptop.

VR porn is more costly than 2D porn, since you must buy a headset. Still, it is growing in popularity. In fact, it is the fastest-growing sector of the entire porn industry.[13] Forty-six percent of US men have experienced virtual reality, and 15 percent have tried VR porn, which means one in three men who have tried any form of VR technology have also watched VR porn.

What about women? Sixty-eight percent of VR headset owners report having watched porn at some point (74 percent of male owners and 57 percent of female owners) and 60 percent of VR headset owners report watching VR porn at least *once per week* (65 percent of male owners and 47 percent of female owners). VR porn is mainly a US market at present. It is currently valued at $1.52 billion and is expected to grow to $124.5 billion by 2030! So if you are a fan of tech or looking for a super realistic and private erotic experience, consider buying some virtual reality goggles for you or your partner and embark on a VR porn adventure alone or together!

I hope that was a pretty fun chapter to read. You should feel as if you have just completed a master class in female sexuality. From the history of erotic imagery to the futuristic immersive experience of VR porn, we have traveled the gamut of erotica throughout time. We have also covered the nuts and bolts of sex aids from lubes to toys.

Now what are you going to do with all that knowledge? Go forth and have fun!

Chapter 10

Other Bedroom Gaps

This book has dealt with the difference in sexual baggage, sexual expectations, and sometimes sexual capabilities between heterosexual, able-bodied, healthy couples in midlife. But the Bedroom Gap applies to a whole lot of us, probably to all of us, albeit in unique ways. The intersectional ageism, sexism, ableism, and homophobia of our era creates ignorance, fear, and myopic views of how sex should "be." Let's remember that the Bedroom Gap—the differences in expectations and abilities between sex partners—is truly a universal issue, and it merits acknowledging a few of the unique versions of the gap out there.

In this chapter we will look at under the radar groups whose Bedroom Gaps might have particular qualities and require particular solutions—but who also crave, need, and enjoy sex as much as anyone.

LGBTQIA+

The LGBTQIA+ population is no stranger to sexual issues; because of stigma and shame, many LGBTQIA+ people don't bring up issues with clinicians or anyone else. But the Bedroom Gap exists in this population as well. For example, the feeling of having to have sex to please a partner, as well as different levels of libido, exists in gay relationships every bit as much as straight ones. Sloane and Lucy are a lesbian couple who see me as patients. They recently came in, frustrated. Sloane has a higher baseline libido than Lucy, who is now also caring for an unwell aging parent and has really stopped engaging sexually with Sloane. Lucy never really cared for sex to begin with, and her history of sexual abuse as a teen by her mother's boyfriend led to sexual aversions that she and I have been working to overcome. Now she is focused on eldercare and is even less interested in an active sex life. The same Bedroom Gap principles apply here: communication in a nonjudgmental way, patience, support, and maybe swapping out hot heavy sex for cuddling, stroking, showering, and naked time. At least for a while.

Lesbian Sex Issues

Lesbians report greater satisfaction with sex, including more and better orgasms than their heterosexual X,X counterparts. Nonetheless, lesbians have a lot in common in terms of sexual dysfunction with heterosexual women; for both groups, the most common issue is hypoactive sexual desire disorder. Causes for HSDD are the same for homosexual and heterosexual women: stressors, work schedule, young children in the home, and sexual abuse or assault history.

Three issues lesbians face that could be distinct from those faced by heterosexual women include:

1. **Internalized and externalized homophobia:** Experiencing homophobia in one's daily life may contribute to

chronic stress. The minority stress model posits that people in minority groups (including ethnic, racial, gender, and sexual minorities and other stigmatized social groups) experience more chronic stress due to societal and cultural discrimination and prejudice. Keep this in mind as you read this chapter. The stress of concealing one's sexuality or "being in the closet" can contribute not only to dysfunction in one's sexual life but also to depression and anxiety disorders that health care providers need to be sensitive to. Despite having higher rates of orgasm and satisfying sex than heterosexual women, lesbian women also report higher rates of anxiety, depression, alcohol and drug use, and sexual dysfunction.

2. **Lesbian connectedness:** Question: What does a lesbian bring on a second date? Answer: a U-Haul. This joke is well known in LGBTQIA+ circles. It makes fun of the eagerness with which lesbians seem to fall hard and form deep attachments to their partners. This can play a role in female sexual dysfunction (FSD) because, not unlike her straight gal pals and their male partners, the lesbian partner must fill more than just the role of tantalizing lover; she must also be stable, loving, and empathic. Recall from Chapter 3 how the relationship therapist Esther Perel pointed out the perils of trying to be too many things in one relationship.

3. **Lesbian bed death:** This misleading and false term refers to the decrease in frequency of sex among lesbian couples in a committed and prolonged relationship. Studies show a drop-off in sexual activity that occurs about two years into long-term lesbian relationships, but this

happens in all long-term sexual relationships, making it not unique to lesbians.[1]

My cousin Lonnie, a proud and sexually active lesbian, tells me, "Lesbians have really hot sex, and they can have really good sex lives well into older age; the stereotype of the doddering lesbian couple knitting scarves and drinking tea together is really outdated; maybe it makes mainstream folks more comfortable than picturing two women having multiple-orgasm sex. Maybe it is easier to imagine that after a certain age, women just are companions and cuddle and hold hands," she shares. (Clearly, this is homophobia, ageism, and sexism all "knitted" together!)

Lonnie continued, "Lesbians are enjoying being able to be out more comfortably, in certain communities at least. We can shop for sex toys in female-forward sex shops. We can find lube and toys for sale even in our local drugstore, and of course there is a lot available online, which is a more private way to amp up lesbian sex life, whether it is sexual aids, BDSM hardware, toys, or lube. And the sex toys on the market today are finally designed for female pleasure, not to mimic a hard penis. We can find visual or audio porn that caters to lesbian tastes. Lesbian porn and female-directed and -created porn are more accessible."

Lonnie paints a fetching picture of lesbian sex life, but she is well aware that despite more openness and acceptance of LGBTQIA+ people, in many communities and countries, religious and political persecution of gay humans has not decreased and in some it seems to be ramping up. But overall, in the privacy of one's own bedroom, better options exist for a robust sex life for lesbians, and a long-lasting one too!

Lonnie has other caveats for this community, however. "Having said that," she goes on, "a lesbian couple going through menopause can be tricky, because if you are both experiencing mood swings, easy crying, anxiety, depression, vaginal dryness, pain with inserting sex toys, it is hard to support each other. At least you get what the other is going through, but you are both struggling."

Trans Women

My practice is half an hour from one of the nation's top transgender surgeons, so I see a lot of transgender women with neovaginas. These are made from a variety of "skin" sources; penile and scrotal skin, as well as extra-genital tissue like peritoneum, intestine, urethral, or oral mucosa, can be used to create a vagina. In gender-affirming vagino-plasty (GAV), the penis is disassembled and a vulva and vagina are constructed from the disassembled parts; because the neovagina is made from tissue that lacks the elasticity and rugae (ridges) of vaginal tissue, the neovagina is intentionally made a bit longer than a natural vagina.[2] Nonetheless, penetrative sex with a neovagina can be quite painful. Remember the Beautiful and Sexy Bartholins's and Skene's glands from Chapter 1, which make our natural lube? Neovaginas lack these glands as well. Pelvic floor physical therapists and I work with my trans women patients to stretch and dilate the tissue but elimination of sexual pain with penetration is challenging.

Trans Men

These patients often have facial and body hair and male musculature thanks to androgen therapy, but many choose to retain their female internal and external genitalia. For trans men, there is a real need for contraception if they have a male partner and PIV sex is part of the sexual repertoire. Trans men also still need HPV vaccination, pap smears, STI screening, and management of pain and bleeding related to periods. They may need IUD insertion or even a hysterectomy. Trans men can find it challenging to live with male gender expression

and outward male appearance but still suffer the indignities of menstruation and the cancer risks that come with female genitalia. This
can create a Bedroom Gap replete with self-loathing, depression, and
myriad sexual issues.

Cancer Survivors

A cancer diagnosis can be devastating, and the *sexual effects* of cancer treatment are often not discussed by doctors (who, again, lack
proper training, are time pressed, might feel it is not their concern,
and bring their own discomfort or prejudices about sex into the exam
room). While the trend in oncology is not just to prolong life but to
maintain *quality of life*, sexual health is often not addressed. So many
of the women I see after a personal or partner's cancer diagnosis feel
ashamed to bring up the topic of sex. Some have been told by their
doctors "you are lucky to be alive!" or "my job is to get rid of the cancer, so let's focus on that." Patients don't know if it is even appropriate
to ask about whether and when and how they can rebuild a sex life.

Since sexual health is part of overall human health, I'd like to give
you cancer survivors and thrivers out there permission to want it, to ask
for it, to get it, to enjoy it. On your own terms, of course. Why should
cancer destroy a part of your life that brings joy, fosters intimacy and
support, and releases neurochemicals that reduce depression?

Breast Cancer

There are over four million breast cancer survivors in the United
States today. Some women diagnosed with breast cancer suffer from
the same feelings that many cancer-diagnosed humans endure—they
feel unwanted, unattractive, less of a woman, especially those women
who undergo mastectomy with or without breast reconstruction surgery. Even women who undergo a "nipple-sparing" lumpectomy can

lose sensation in the nipple. And like prostate cancer patients, some breast cancer patients take hormone-blocking medications such as tamoxifen and aromatase inhibitors to reduce recurrence rates. While these anti-estrogen medications have been a godsend—showing a 30 percent reduction in breast cancer recurrence—they wreak havoc on genital tissues, which are estrogen and testosterone dependent. These medications basically accelerate the development of GSM (remember from Chapter 1, GSM is the loss of moisture, blood vessels, and collagen that comes from lack of estrogen), so a forty-five-year-old with breast cancer on an aromatase inhibitor for five or ten years might have the vagina of a seventy-year-old!

Breast cancer patients on anti-estrogen medications often come to my office in tears. "Look, I'm grateful to be alive, but I had no idea that these medications would destroy my sex life," Talia tells me. "The medications are life prolonging, I know, but they sapped all the health from my vagina; it feels dry as a desert, like my vagina is made of sandpaper, and there is no way, just no way, to have sex." Others feel angry that they weren't warned of the sexual fallout: "Nobody mentioned to me that this would happen. In some ways, losing my vaginal health and my sexual capacity has been harder on me and on my marriage than the cancer itself," one patient confided.

In the name of curing disease and maintaining the aesthetics of a normal female shape, breasts are "surgerized," irradiated, stuffed with implants, nipple tattooed, and rebuilt. Even these quality-of-life advances in cancer care are cause for anxiety and tears, micro indignities of disease, and things to explain to sex partners.

Gynecologic Cancers

These cancers—ovarian, uterine, vulvar, and cervical—may not be treated with anti-estrogen meds but can destroy a sex life simply because the surgeries can be so destructive to female anatomy. I was speaking at a women's event last year, and after the event I was swarmed with women asking questions, sharing stories, the usual. One woman quietly handed me a slip of paper with "vulvar cancer, please help me" and her phone number.

The next week as I examined her, I had to admit there was little I could do for her: The scarring from her surgery and radiation had left her vaginal opening the diameter of a pencil. The labia minora were gone, the clitoris covered over with a dense, whitish scar. Even my go-to cure-all, vaginal estrogen, would be of little use. There was very little vascularized tissue left to respond to the estrogen.

Lorrie is a petite actress in her late thirties from New York, with a pixie haircut and a lot of spunk. She is actively online dating, but the surgery and radiation from her cervical cancer has made penetrative sex all but impossible. "The guys I date want sex, and they want kids, and when I tell them I have no uterus and a vagina as stiff as a lead pipe," she animatedly tells me, "they mostly don't go for a second date. It's just a deal-breaker."

Surgery can destroy the vagina and the vulva, including the labia and/or the clitoris. Inside the abdomen and pelvis, scarring can lead to chronic pain. Radiation to the pelvis can render vaginal tissue white, stiff, and nearly devoid of sensation, and sex can be incredibly painful. My advice: Sex can also be a part of the emotional if not physical part of healing from cancer. Don't give up on it, but be patient, accept that you may never get back to your precancer sex life, keep humor present, and find new ways to enjoy what your new anatomy allows. Consider working with a pelvic floor physical therapist, who can help with pain, dilator use, and relaxation techniques. Consider surgical reconstruction if possible. Also seek out clinicians who proactively address the sexual side effects before your surgery or radiation therapy, so you are prepared and feel your clinician is committed to your overall wellness, including your sex life.

Prostate Cancer

One of my friends, Lindsey, sixty-two, shared the conflicted emotions surrounding the sexual effects of her husband's prostate cancer. "When we were told that Jamey had prostate cancer, and that he would need prostate surgery, which would mean the end of sex as we knew it, Jamey cried, but I felt this burden, the burden of marital obligation to have sex, relieved of me. Then I felt guilty about that. I knew we as a couple would have to create a new definition of sex. We still have sex, but it is different. In some ways it is better because we can be friendly, funny, intimate, without the expectation of penetration and orgasm."

Bedroom Gaps after prostate surgery are common and devastating. Prostate cancer surgery (prostatectomy, or removal of the prostate) can have dramatic changes for a man's sex life. The nerves responsible for erections can be damaged by prostate surgery, and so the majority of the 3.3 million prostate cancer survivors in the United States today have erectile dysfunction. What's more, ED can be made worse by medications taken for cancer or for other reasons.

The good news is that help is available in various ways, including:

- Oral medications such as Viagra, Levitra, Cialis[3]
- VED: Vacuum erection device pumps
- Injections of alprostadil, a prostaglandin that causes vasodilation and facilitates erection
- MUSE intraurethral prostaglandin gel

Oral medications only help about 50 percent of the time, according to sexuality counselor and author Anne Katz. Katz points out that "for the first two years after prostate surgery, erections may improve on their own, but improvement usually maxes out after 2 years."[4] It is easy to see why prostate cancer is a setup for a Bedroom Gap, especially since the mean age for prostate cancer diagnosis is sixty-seven and most women by this age have pretty severe GSM. Amazingly, orgasms are still possible for men after prostate surgery, even with a flaccid penis, and are sometimes more intense, sometimes less, than before surgery. What is not possible after prostatectomy is ejaculation because the fluid part of the ejaculate is made in the prostate. On top of that, the penis is about an inch shorter after prostate surgery, drawn in to the abdomen when the prostate is removed; for men already insecure about penile length this can be an issue. Not only the length but the stability of the penis is reduced with prostate surgery; missionary position might not really be possible and side-by-side or rear entry usually works better because penetration can be accomplished more easily with a prostate-less penis that lacks support.[5]

And just as breast cancer treatment may involve surgery and long-term medication to prevent recurrence, prostate cancer may also involve hormone-blocking medications after surgery. Anti-androgen therapy, which blocks the production of androgens such as testosterone, is used as treatment in some prostate cancers and is analogous to anti-estrogen therapy for some breast cancers. Blocking androgens can have dramatic side effects that impact a man's sex life, including lowering libido, ED, mood swings, weight gain, hot flashes, loss of muscle mass and strength, and gynecomastia, the development of breast tissue. Men feel ashamed, embarrassed, less "masculine." Many of these symptoms mirror the miserable menopausal symptoms women face. Libido is not directly affected by removal of the prostate, but some men may feel less interest in sex if ejaculation is absent and erections are problematic.

Surgical, Chemical, or Immunological Menopause

One of my patients, Cailey, talked to me about the issues of chemically induced menopause, in which a woman is going through this difficult life phase far before she or her friends have started talking about such things: "I am thirty-six but my ovaries stopped when I was twenty-three. I have such bad vaginal dryness, my partner can't use his fingers, a dildo, and no way a penis. I understood that my fertility was compromised, but not that I would be needing lube my whole life and that sex would suffer so severely and so soon."

If a woman has her ovaries removed surgically, or ovarian function is destroyed immunologically from premature ovarian insufficiency (POI) or radiation or chemotherapy, menopause and its sexual side effects can develop more abruptly and more severely than in women who undergo menopause naturally. POI patients need HT to prevent the widespread deterioration of bones, heart, and brain seen in menopause but also to keep their genitourinary tract healthy. Far too few clinicians understand this. If you have POI do not wait for a physician to tell you that you need HT. Seek it out yourself and don't forget that vaginal health is urinary and sexual health as well.

Chronic Illness

Some men and women with cancer want very much to work at maintaining a sex life as a way to move past a cancer diagnosis and a way to feel alive, as a fully functioning human being, rather than as a cancer survivor or a diagnosis. So do people with chronic illnesses, such as diabetes and cardiovascular disease.

My uncle, Sophocles M. Sophocles, was a character. Born in Cyprus, he came to the United States as a rambunctious boy. He married, had two children, and lived an interesting life as a priest, artist, author, and philosopher. He had two PhDs, was a Fulbright scholar, a university professor, and a beloved member of his community. He wore a beret, drove a Thunderbird, had a Thoreau-level love of nature, and loved to smoke, which contributed to his premature heart disease. He eschewed traditional medical care and opted for supplements suggested by someone peddling "natural remedies" for his chest pains. Uncle Soph had his first heart attack at thirty-nine and then a fatal heart attack at fifty-eight, during sex. His wife, Chrysanthe, lived another forty-two years and, perhaps less inhibited in her late nineties, told me, "We were having sex on the living room floor of our beach house. I was on top, which we liked, and he just got chest pain and passed out and the paramedics couldn't revive him. After he died, I decided just to please myself sexually and not to remarry, because I love sex and I didn't want to worry that I would give another man a heart attack. Two sex deaths were more than I wanted on my resume." While I miss my charismatic, brilliant uncle who left us too soon, I love that my Aunt Chris defined pleasure on her own terms after her husband's death, and I respect that she prioritized it in her life and embraced solo pleasure for the four decades she remained alive as a widow.

Bedroom Gaps for people with chronic illness pose their own set of issues, which can be an added burden on top of Bedroom Gap issues related to aging or communication. Chronic conditions such as diabetes and heart disease can ruin a sex life, especially after a heart attack or stroke. For example, diabetes, which affects nearly forty million people in the United States, destroys small blood vessels and can cause erectile issues for men and yeast infections for women.[6] People are often afraid to have sex after a heart attack, and their partners are afraid the sex will trigger another cardiac event.

As a rule of thumb, if your heart is strong enough to tolerate a brisk walk or climbing a flight of stairs, you can resume sexual activity. Obviously, this depends on when and whether you are cleared to resume sex by your doctor and on the severity of the heart attack and whether you also have congestive heart failure or abnormal heart rhythms, which may preclude sexual activity. Ready to try after a heart attack? Start slowly and set yourself up for success, meaning don't have sex in positions that put pressure on your chest, don't have sex after a meal since your stomach needs the blood flow for digestion, avoid sex after drinking alcohol since it can make erections harder to attain and to maintain and can decrease genital sensation for women. You also may need nitroglycerine or other medications before sex to improve cardiac blood flow.[7] These are general guidelines and suggestions and are not a substitute for personalized medical advice from your doctor. The National Cancer Institute (cancer.gov), the American Heart Association (heart.org), and the American Cancer Society (cancer.org) all have booklets about sex and illness as places to start.

As with all Bedroom Gaps, help to overcome the one widened or caused by a cancer diagnosis or chronic illness relies on open communication. If you are a cancer survivor or had a recent heart attack, know that your partner is worried about how to broach the subject, feeling it might appear selfish. He/she might worry that having sex could cause another heart event, or cause your cancer to recur, or cause a new cancer to develop, or spread cancer left behind. If your partner has health issues, be an informed part of his/her treatment and healing so you can know when you would likely be able to resume sex, and in what way. What are the limitations and changes, and how can you reinvent your sex life within the confines of these limitations? Cancer and chronic illness don't have to cause or widen a Bedroom Gap—but it will require some effort and creativity and perhaps a dash of humor to keep things healthy in the bedroom during health struggles like these.

Disability

When we think of sex, we think of a young, fit, healthy cisgender man and woman, not unlike what Hollywood spoon-feeds us over and over. We don't picture morbidly obese, or post–heart attack, or post-chemotherapy patients having sex. We don't think about people with arthritis and hip replacements, much less with ostomies, prosthetics, amputations. We don't think of people with autism spectrum disorder (ASD) or Down syndrome. We literally can't even picture it, or don't want to. Remember the minority stress model discussed previously? It is easier for the collective "we" to assume this crowd is asexual or just doesn't have sex.[8] The Bedroom Gap for disabled people, whether the disability involves one partner or both, is gaping indeed. And, according to the Centers of Disease Control, there are sixty-one million (physically or mentally) disabled Americans today.[9] The pervasive belief that disabled people are asexual means they are left out of the conversation and omitted from information about sexual norms, sexual trends, STI outbreaks, and overall knowledge and education about sex compared with nondisabled peers. This leaves them vulnerable to sexual exploitation, nonconsensual experiences, and overall "bad sex."[10] What's worse, health care providers also don't think of disabled people as sexual beings and are less inclined to ask about sexual health in a disabled patient.[11] This is a big, giant Bedroom Gap.

Okay, but for those of you who are disabled and want to have sex, how do you do it? An appendix at the end of the book shares sex positions and explanations that can improve the experience for people with disabilities. And check out chronicsex.org for a super inclusive website whose mission is "to open up frank discussions and ruminations about how quality of life is affected [in people with chronic illness and disability]," specifically focusing on self-love, self-care, relationships, sexuality, and sex itself.[12]

The largest group of Americans with disabilities are those 35.5 million Americans with cognitive disabilities, including 6 million people with autism (ASD). Autism is more prevalent in men, but women with autism may be underdiagnosed or diagnosed later in life. Bedroom Gaps among autistic couples or in cases where one partner is on the autism spectrum arise from challenges with (1) communication, (2) social interaction, (3) misinterpretation of social cues and boundaries, (4) sensory processing issues, and (5) lack of sex education because the community believes autistic individuals are asexual. The lack of sex ed can lead to lack of information about consent or pregnancy or STI prevention and increased risk of sexual victimization. There are increased rates of gender dysphoria and non-heterosexual orientation (asexuality, bisexuality, homosexuality) among those with ASD. Sex education for adolescents and clinicians alike should include specialized information for those with cognitive disabilities, so that both clinicians and patients can be comfortable discussing sex and be cognizant of particular issues. The 60 million plus disabled Americans have the same right to bodily autonomy and sexual pleasure as everyone else.[13]

Senior Sex and the Bedroom Gap

We are living longer, staying healthier longer, and wanting to stay sexually active longer, and this is great! But it means that the Bedroom Gap of midlife sex has a geriatric counterpart that must be addressed. See, not only does nobody teach us what happens to our sexual selves in midlife, but *noooobody* talks about sex in the latter decades of life. Remember, being alive after sixty-five is a relatively new thing in a human evolutionary sense, since for most of human history, we didn't live long enough to worry about what sex would be like after our reproductive potential ended.[14] But our species is living longer, especially in the developed world.

From 2022 to 2050, the over-sixty-five population in the United States is expected to increase from 57.8 million to 82 million.[15] The Census Bureau projects that the number of people over ninety and over one hundred will quadruple from 2024 to 2054.[16] There are currently about 2 million American nonagenarians and one hundred thousand centenarians. So, yes, the over-sixty-five population is growing, is sexually active, and is living a lot longer.

Sex . . . at My Age?

You bet! The University of Michigan's National Poll on Healthy Aging in 2018 shed light on sexual interests and habits of sixty-five to eighty-year-olds. On average, 65 percent of this cohort is interested in sex, 40 percent are sexually active, and 73 percent of those sexually active are sexually satisfied.[17] This is great news, meaning that the Bedroom Gaps of midlife, and honestly the biases of media and sex ed, that set us up for Bedroom Gaps right from our earliest days of sex, seem to close with advanced age. Perhaps there is an acceptance of our limitations, an awareness of our mortality, an ability to focus on the joy of whatever version of sex we can muster, and a pleasure in sex as a means to intimacy and human connectivity. Seventy-six percent of respondents in the healthy aging poll felt sex was an important part of a romantic relationship. Fifty-four percent said sex is an important component to overall quality of life. Wonderfully, these numbers did not decrease with increasing age groups in the study.[18] If you are reading this book and you are over sixty-five, these numbers should be encouraging to you. *You have a right to sexual pleasure at any age*, even if mainstream media neglects to portray this and doctors discount sex as part of your overall health.

Alone with Our Bodies, Ourselves

Women in general outlive men, and the census data also shows there *are more older women living alone.* As of 2023, over a quarter of women ages sixty-five to seventy-four live alone, as do 39 percent of women ages seventy-five to eighty-four and fully half of women over age eighty-five.[19] Remember that staying sexually active contributes to overall health and reduced depression. Let me leave you with an encouraging quote from the PhD sexologist Betty Dodson:

> The decade of my seventies, which I see as the youth of old age, was far more delightful than I could have imagined. It was some of the best partner sex ever. . . . Now . . . at eighty-one . . . I can still walk, talk, laugh, sing, dance, write, and have an orgasm any time I desire with one of my many vibrators and a fantasy. . . . I prefer to see death as my final work of art, the ultimate orgasm being when the life force leaves my body. Until then, I'll continue to figure out ways to enjoy my older body. As long as I can access my mind for sexual memories and fantasies while I hold a vibrator on my clitoris for one more orgasm, I'm here for the long haul as I head for one hundred or more.[20]

Conclusion

The Bedroom Gap is real. In my thirty years of clinical practice, talking with and listening to women and men, a few things have become apparent:

- **The Bedroom Gap is ubiquitous**—when I started writing this book, I was focused on the Bedroom Gap as a problem for menopausal women with GSM. But what is now so obvious to me is that the Bedroom Gap is so much bigger than GSM and menopause-related issues. The Bedroom Gap applies to women of all ages, across a broad spectrum of religious, cultural, gender, and sexual identities.
- **The Bedroom Gap is a product of huge forces**, including
  - **Time Honed Gender Bias:** Millennia of patriarchal rules and sexual scripts control the sexual narrative of what is sex, what is good sex, who gets to have pleasure, and what is the role of women in heterosexual sex.
  - **Big Porn:** The power of porn to teach us what heterosexual women should be doing, what men want, is massive, pervasive, and destructive. It has led us to sex that trends toward coercion, physicality, demeaning behavior toward women, entitlement, intimate partner violence, assault, and rape. It has also misled men and women in terms of

what is a healthy way to have sex. We need to uproot the misogyny in porn and shift to a pleasure-focused rather than a (male) orgasm-focused sexual experience.

- **Big Pharma and Big Tech:** Scientific research and development has shifted from the campus to the corporate. The US government has historically been a large source of funding for all scientific research, but as of 2025 there has been an assault on the US scientific community, the downstream effects of which are hard to calculate. What predated this scientific maelstrom and what will likely remain a bane to progress in sexual health solutions is the profound discrepancy in funding for clinical research on male versus female issues, including sexual health. The Bedroom Gap will never close if we don't develop clinical solutions to problems relating to menopause and the loss of ovarian estrogen; if we don't fund tech companies that offer sexual wellness solutions for women; and unless we stop thinking of women past their reproductive age as societally worth less than their younger peers.

- **Negligent Medical Education System:** Until we teach what really happens to women's bodies throughout their lifespan and step out from the shadows of shame and ignorance about basic anatomy and physiology, our clinicians will remain inadequately trained to help women with issues related to ovarian aging and sex, and they will not be open to or able to help their patients with Bedroom Gap issues.

- **Sex Education:** A provincial and fear-based approach to sex education is forcing our youth to rely on porn as their most available teacher of sex and, worse, of human relations. Sex ed should be progressive and pleasure and consent focused, not fear based.

In this book we have learned about female sexual function and about how to enjoy sex at any age. We have shared ways for you to privately improve your sexual experience, foster intimacy, and prioritize pleasure. But never forget that the enormous gender inequality in health care, including sexual health care, needs more than just you closing your own Bedroom Gap.

It requires exposure of the inequities in teaching; it requires upending sex ed, the medical education system, the biopharma industry, and the venture capital firms that fund the startups of today. It involves embracing and supporting a new kind of female-forward porn, so that the unsafe side of porn, the exploitation of children, and the gender-demeaning aspects of the genre can be replaced with ethical, respectful filming with consideration of the female gaze.

We decry sex as shameful, dirty; we keep it hidden; we don't talk about it. We pretend we don't see it, don't need it, but we all do it. These falsely conservative values do not serve us. They simply add to the irony of our sexual secrecy. We allow and applaud machismo, sexist comments and behaviors, not to mention positive portrayals of womanizers, lotharios, and alpha males in media, but we are afraid to publicly support healthy sexual values (including intimacy and female pleasure, not to mention the sexiness of reproductive rights and reliable contraception). The messages this sends to women are damaging!

When we herald submissive, male orgasm–focused porn, we send women the message: Pleasure is not for you. When we ban a congresswoman for using the word *vagina* and promote unattainable beauty standards for female genitals, we send women a message: Be ashamed of your anatomy. When we reduce a woman's right to reproductive health, contraceptive access, and the choice of when to be pregnant, we send a message: Others control your body, and your life. When we don't prosecute a sexual predator, or let him off easy, we send a message that it is partly the victim's fault and that men are entitled to a woman's body, whether with or without consent. Believe it or not, all of these relate to the Bedroom Gap. They all play into the thoughts, fears, shame, expectations, misgivings, frustrations, and actions a woman brings to her bedroom life, and to her role in that room.

So I invite you, now, to take a look around your own bedroom. Look at the bed. Think about what it represents, and about the woman you want to bring there. A woman brimming with confidence, pride, joy, humor, and curiosity. A woman knowledgeable about her body and who has given herself permission to have pleasure be part of her due. Whatever your assigned or identified gender, ask yourself, "Is this the bedroom I want? Am I doing my gender justice in accepting the status quo?" If not, I invite you to reflect on how it could be better, and how you, in your own singular way, can close your Bedroom Gap and move the gender equality needle ever so slightly forward. And by the way, if you are truly happy, truly satisfied, truly cool with your level of sexual satisfaction, then pass this book on to someone who might have some room to grow.

I am in New York tonight seeing a play at Lincoln Center. As I walk past the center's glass-walled restaurant, I am reminded of the serendipitous encounter with Gloria Steinem in the coat closet; of the mandate she leveled at me that night to write this book. I have grown so much in writing it that in reading the introduction again, that piece of writing and that closet encounter with Gloria seem a long time ago, a journey ago. It is odd, but the idea of this book began as a way for me to share thirty years of medical expertise; it turns out that the teacher was a student and that the endeavor has been its own learning journey for me as a doctor, a woman, a mother, and a feminist. Thanks for joining me.

Acknowledgments

Thank you to Gloria Steinem, for inspiration and an honest talk in a coat closet; Ruth Westheimer, for advice and aspiration delivered with zest; Kate Manne, for letting me audit your class and hear your humble brilliance; Michelle Toth, for guiding my beginning; Amaryah Orenstein, for holding my hand from proposal to publication; Laurel Braitman, for saying "Yes, you can;" Diana Ventimiglia, the team at Hachette, and Jane Fransson, for walking with me through the chapters and the process; Brad and Suzy Ginsberg, who believed a long time ago; and, to Sarah Hall Productions, for believing now.

Thank you also:

To my Besties: Loretta, Lorraine, Leslie, Rebecca, Nina, Tory, and Bruce.

To my Dear Ones: Aris, Ros, Jo, Kate and Amy, Despy, Chrysanthe, Maria Samara, Maria L, Kelly, Vibha, Catherine, Amy, Aia, Robin, Laura, Melissa, Julie, Bunny, Allegra, Piraye, Mara, Diane, Evonne, Emer, Brian, Nathan, Muredach, Paul and Mark, Simba, Rikke, Mireia, Jenny McC, Barrie, Jennifer BL, Lanniece, Leslie O-T, SonoMamma, Dina; HBS Forum 23; the AIS sisters; and the Princeton gang: Jill, Nancy, Sharon, Whitney, Mollie, Vicky, Lynne, Elizabeth.

To the Women's Healthcare of Princeton family, for supporting progressive medicine and creating a space where women feel heard and dignified.

To a singular humanitarian, Dr. Faiza Sadiq. Your loyalty, intelligence, and friendship move and inspire me. Love you more, my friend.

To the team at TED who believed the Bedroom Gap was a universal message.

To my MenoSphere, including the Menopause Mafia, the MenoPosse, and my mentors Jim Simon, Wen Shen, Andrew Goldstein, Sheryl Kingsberg, Irwin Goldstein, Risa Kagan, Mary Jane Minkin, Diana Bitner, Susan Spadt, Mike Ingber, Daniel Soffer, Dan Rader, and Paul Grewal. Also to Jen Eident, Katie Fogarty, and Jen Weiss-Wolf; Joanna, Jill, Kathleen, and Mindy at Midi; to Let's Talk Menopause, Liz and Heather at EMBR Labs, and the SheMedia team.

To the Hotties: Kristi, Kerry, Cathy, Gabriella Lina, and Zameer for believing that sex in midlife was worthy of a documentary.

To the Humenotarians: Charles and Ben Odipo and the Friends of Yimbo; and to Bea Dixon, Ali Savaya, and the Honey Pot family.

To Senator Shirley Turner and the indefatigable reproductive rights activist nonagenarian Suzy Wilson for never ever ever giving up the fight for women in New Jersey.

To the spectacular educators who nurtured my love affair with words and writing, from The Tarleton School and Westtown Friends School to The Agnes Irwin School and Duke University. A lucky girl indeed.

To my extended MartinCyrusSophocles family, whose love and support was always there, especially my favorite (and only) sister.

To Thomas Siomporas and Michael and Despina Sophocles, who left Greece a century ago with their only certainty being their integrity, intellect, grit, and love of family, for the uncertainty of life, and the opportunity for education in the United States.

Appendix One

❧

Sex Positions for People with Disabilities

See the link in the endnotes from Ro.com, where you'll find stick figures of the positions described in this appendix.[1]

1. Modified Missionary

This position leaves the bottom partner's hands free to explore the standing partner's erogenous zones.

Instructions:

- The partner with limited mobility lays on the bed with their butt on the edge.
- The other partner stands between their legs, facing the bed.
- The standing partner lifts their partner's legs so their ankles are resting on their shoulders.
- Alternatively, the partner with limited mobility can rest their legs on a chair behind the standing partner.

Who benefits?

- Couples in which one person has limited mobility and the other doesn't
- If either or both partners have obesity
- People with an ostomy bag (a pouch affixed to the abdomen to collect stool, often needed after certain bowel surgeries)
- Pregnant women

2. Face-to-Face

This position allows for face-to-face intimacy.

Instructions:

- The partner with limited mobility sits in a chair, a wheel-chair with armrests removed, or on the edge of the bed.
- Their partner straddles them and wraps their arms around them.
- The partner on top braces their feet on the edge of the bed to thrust.
- The partner on the bed can assist by grabbing their partner's buttocks and lifting and bouncing.

Who benefits?

- People with limited mobility
- People who have muscle spasms when lying down
- People with chronic fatigue

3. Intimate Sitting

This position gives control to the top partner if the other has limited mobility.

Instructions:

- The partner with limited mobility sits on the bed with their legs outstretched. Placing pillows behind the back or resting against the headboard may make this position more comfortable.
- The other partner straddles their waist, puts their feet on the bed, and then bends their knees to lower down.

Who benefits?

- Those looking for face-to-face intimacy
- Couples in which one partner has limited mobility and the other does not

4. Spooning or Side-Lying

This position allows both partners to have their hands free to stimulate other areas. Spooning is great for people with conditions like arthritis, and the bed absorbs pressure on the joints.

Instructions:

- Both partners lay on their sides facing the same direction.
- Alternatively, one partner can wrap their top leg over the other partner's thigh to help support each other in the position.

Who benefits?

- Pregnant women
- If either or both partners have obesity
- People with lower back pain, arthritis, and chronic pain

5. Modified Doggy-Style Position #1
This position is helpful if using a wheelchair and more comfortable for those with joint pain.

Instructions:
- The partner with limited mobility moves their wheelchair to the edge of the bed or sits in a chair.
- The other partner lowers themselves on top of the bottom partner, so their back faces the other partner's stomach.
- The person on top rests their arms and upper body on the bed while thrusting.

Who benefits?
- One wheelchair-bound partner and one partner without disability
- People with hip pain

6. Modified Doggy-Style Position #2
This position allows for a head-to-toe physical connection.

Instructions:
- Arrange a few pillows on the floor or bed to support the partner with limited mobility.
- The other partner lies on top, with their chest against the back of the lower partner.

Who benefits?
- People who require more stability as the bottom partner

7. Sideways 69

This position leaves both people free to stimulate each other with their fingers, tongue, or sex toys.

Instructions:
- One partner lies on their side in the spooning position.
- The other partner lays facing them with their head at the opposite end.

Who benefits?
- People with weak or spastic hips
- People with arthritis or fragile joints

Appendix Two

Podcasts, Porn Sites, Oh My

Below is a list of various podcasts and websites that can help you on your path to understanding and getting more comfortable with your sexuality and bring you closer to the kind of pleasure you desire and deserve.

Some Porn Sites Built for Women:
- Lust Cinema
- MakeLoveNotPorn
- The Crash Pad
- Lady Cheeky
- Dame Jones
- Indie Porn Revolution

Audio Porn Sites to Check Out[1]
- Quinn: This easy-to-use app lets you choose stories to listen to.
- Dipsea: A huge library of short sex stories; also guided erotic exercises.

- Tumblr: User-submitted clips, including direct-to-listener clips where the narrator speaks directly to you the listener; also blogs.
- Audible: This is a site for audiobooks, but you can search "erotic" to have someone read sexy content to you.
- Scribd: Ditto.
- Literotica: Over thirty different categories; user-written stories.
- Bellesa: Includes bisexual and nonbinary categories.
- Bust: "One handed Reads"—I love this image! These are nine-hundred-word stories that will get your juices flowing.
- Girl on the net: UK-based sex blogger's audio site.
- Vibease: Sells original audio erotica and sex toys for purchase as well as tips on masturbation. Note: Some of their Bluetooth toys will link to some stories on this site.
- Reddit: Subreddits: gonewildaudio, pillowtalkaudio. Note: You can post requests that others on Reddit can fill.
- Audio Desires—Sexy stories also in other languages.

If You Are More the Podcast Type, Here Are Some Beloved Erotic Podcasts:
- Fangasm: Erotic fan fiction, seriously. Who knew you could have sexy thoughts about Harry Potter and Ron Weasley?
- Dirty Diana: Focused on female sexual desires, voice acted by Demi Moore and other known actors.
- Thirst Aid Kit: All about celebrity crushes.
- Bawdy Storytelling: Unscripted stories of sex and body image.
- Probably True: LGBTQ issues presented in a lighthearted but still steamy way by host Scott Flashheart.

- Turn Me On: Modern topics addressed by hosts Jeremie and Bryde (who used to be an item), including kink, polyamory, and dating apps.
- Sex with Strangers: International and intersectional perspectives on sexuality and sex.
- Where Should We Begin: Esther Perel lets us sit in on real couples' therapy sessions.
- Savage Lovecast: Dan Savage gives advice on lots of aspects of love and sex.
- Dying for Sex: Host Nikki Boyer talks about how to live fully present in the moment and offers advice on life, death, and sex.
- Sex with Emily: Hosted by sex therapist Dr. Emily Morse; nonjudgmental and informative.
- The Sex Wrap: Answering listeners' questions about all things sex.
- Salty Sex Cast: Breaking down sexual taboos.
- Sexology: Hosted by Dr. Nazarin Moali, explores the psychology of sex.
- The Sex Therapy podcast: Experts and celebrities discuss sex topics.
- The Ultimate Intimacy Podcast: Married couple Nick and Amy host this podcast about sex and intimacy and share personal experiences.
- Better Sex: Hosted by sex therapist Jessa Zimmerman.
- Foreplay Radio: Couples therapist George Faller and sex therapist Dr. Laurie Watson help couples maintain an emotionally connected relationship.
- Call Her Daddy: Alex Cooper gets real and honest on all topics female, dating, relationships, health, and more.

- Brown Girls Do It Too: Conversations about sex in South Asian communities.
- Doing It!: Brit Hannah Witton is open about the challenges of sex with chronic illness, including an ostomy.
- Dying for Sex: Miniseries podcast about a woman with stage 4 breast cancer and the value of friendship.

Notes

Introduction

1. Robinson Meyer and Ashley Fetters, "Victoria-Era Orgasms and the Crisis of Peer Review," *The Atlantic*, September 6, 2018, https://www.theatlantic.com/health/archive/2018/09/victorian-vibrators-orgasms-doctors/569446.
2. Wen Shen, interview by author, November 4, 2024.
3. In 2023 Gloria Steinem noted that we still have a wage gap fifty years after the Equal Pay Act and that closing it in the United States alone would inject $400 billion into the economy! Gloria Steinem, adrienne maree brown, Amanda Nguyen, and Tina Tchen, "Understanding the Wage Gap," MasterClass, accessed August 27, 2025, https://www.masterclass.com/classes/redefining-feminism-with-gloria-steinem-and-noted-co-instructors/chapters/understanding-the-wage-gap.
4. Deepa Narayan, "7 Beliefs That Can Silence Women—and How to Unlearn Them," TED Talks India, May 2019, video available at https://www.ted.com/talks/deepa_narayan_7_beliefs_that_can_silence_women_and_how_to_unlearn_them?subtitle=en.
5. I love words and their etymologies. Here's a good one: "pyrrhic victory," a victory nearly as costly as a defeat. The term comes from the Greek king Pyrrhus of Epirus.
6. Jennifer Weiss-Wolf, "A Citizen's Guide to Menopause Advocacy," Oprah Daily, February 28, 2025, https://www.oprahdaily.com/life/health/a63831343/menopause-advocacy-excerpt-guide/.

Chapter 1: What Happens to Our Lady Bits in Middle Age

1. "Menopause," World Health Organization, October 16, 2024, https://www.who.int/news-room/fact-sheets/detail/menopause#.
2. "quarter of all females": "Menopause," World Health Organization; "60 percent": Kyveli Angelou, Themos Grigoriadis, Michail Diakosavvas, Dimitris Zacharakis, and Stavros Athanasiou, "The Genitourinary Syndrome of Menopause: An Overview of the Recent Data," *Cureus* 12, no. 4 (2020): e7586.

3. Maria Sophocles, "What Happens to Sex in Midlife? A Look at the 'Bedroom Gap,'" TEDWomen, October 2023, video available at https://www.ted.com/talks/maria _sophocles_what_happens_to_sex_in_midlife_a_look_at_the_bedroom_gap ?subtitle=en.

4. A microbiome is basically the microorganisms—viruses and bacteria—that live in a particular part of the body.

5. No judgment here, by the way, with respect to grooming of the genital area. You have every right to wax, laser, shave, depilate, or just go au naturel—whatever you prefer, and it doesn't matter what anyone else thinks. Brooke Shields put it well during a panel on women's health and beauty standards at South by Southwest in 2024, an event we were both speaking at. "You have to be OK going in whatever way feels right to you. If Botox makes you feel good about yourself, do it! If going gray feels right, that's all good, too." But as a doctor, I do like to remind people that pubic hair serves a purpose! Actually several purposes: (1) to protect the delicate vulvar skin from friction and abrasion during sex; (2) to keep germs, dust, and dirt out of the vagina to prevent infection; and (3) to trap sweat, oil, and bacteria in order to keep the vulva and vagina clean (a little odor is normal, that is your pubic hair doing its job). Researchers even suspect pubic hair may play a role in sexual attraction and sexual pleasure. See Holly W. Commings, "To Shave or Not to Shave: An Ob-Gyn's Guide to Pubic Hair Care," American College of Obstetricians and Gynecologists, June 2023, https://www.acog.org/womens-health/experts-and-stories/the-latest/to -shave-or-not-to-shave-an-ob-gyns-guide-to-pubic-hair-care.

6. Shilpa N. Bhupathiraju, Francine Grodstein, Meir J. Stampfer, Walter C. Willett, Carolyn J. Crandall, Jan L. Shifren, et al., "Vaginal Estrogen Use and Chronic Disease Risk in the Nurses' Health Study," *Menopause* 26, no. 6 (2018): 603–610.

7. "Let's Talk About Sex: The Majority of Older Adults Are Satisfied with Their Sex Lives," National Poll on Healthy Aging, Institute for Healthcare Policy and Innovation, University of Michigan, accessed July 16, 2025, https://www .healthyagingpoll.org/reports-more/report/lets-talk-about-sex.

8. Rossella E. Nappi and Marta Kokot-Kierepa, "Vaginal Health: Insights, Views and Attitudes (VIVA)—Results from an International Survey," *Climacteric* 15, no. 1 (2012): 36–44.

Chapter 2: Sex, Sexism, and the Little Blue Pill

1. Elizabeth Selvin, Arthur L. Burnett, and Elizabeth A. Platz, "Prevalence and Risk Factors for Erectile Dysfunction in the US," *American Journal of Medicine* 120, no. 2 (2007:) 151–157.

2. "Pfizer Now Takes Viagra Hoopla to Other Countries," *Advertising Age*, May 3, 1999.

3. See Viagra.com, accessed July 17, 2025.

4. Meika Loe, *The Rise of Viagra: How the Little Blue Pill Changed Sex in America* (New York University Press, 2004), 10.

5.   The answer seems to be yes: ADHD diagnoses have increased across age groups in recent decades. For example, in the UK, between 2000 and 2018 ADHD diagnoses increased approximately twentyfold and prescriptions increased nearly fiftyfold in men between the ages of eighteen and twenty-nine. See Douglas G. J. McKechnie, Elizabeth O'Nions, Sandra Dunsmuir, and Irene Petersen, "Attention-Deficit Hyperactivity Disorder Diagnoses and Prescriptions in UK Primary Care, 2000–2018: Population-Based Cohort Study," *BJPsych Open* 9, no. 4 (2023): e121.

6.   Jami Demuth, "ADHD on TikTok," *Attention Magazine*, August 2002, https://chadd .org/adhd-news/adhd-news-adults/attention-adhd-on-tiktok/.

7.   Christel Renoux, Ju-Young Shin, Sophie Dell'Aniello, Emma Fergusson, and Samy Suissa, "Prescribing Trends of Attention-Deficit Hyperactivity Disorder (ADHD) Medications in UK Primary Care, 1995–2015," *British Journal of Clinical Pharmacology* 82, no. 3 (2016): 858–868; Dawn Connelly, "Special Report: Charting the Rise in ADHD Prescribing," *Pharmaceutical Journal*, July 27, 2023, https://pharmaceutical-journal.com/article/feature/special-report-charting-the-rise -in-adhd-prescribing.

8.   "Worldwide Revenue of Pfizer's Viagra from 2003 to 2019," Statista, accessed August 27, 2008, https://www.statista.com/statistics/264827/pfizers-worldwide -viagra-revenue-since-2003/.

9.   Sameer S. Chopra, "Industry Funding of Clinical Trials: Benefit or Bias?," *JAMA* 290, no. 1 (2003): 113–114.

10. "The State of U.S. Science and Engineering 2020," National Science Board, January 2020, https://ncses.nsf.gov/pubs/nsb20201/u-s-r-d-performance-and-funding.

11. Irwin Goldstein, Arthur L. Burnett, Raymond C. Rosen, Peter W. Park, and Vera J. Stecher, "The Serendipitous Story of Sildenafil: An Unexpected Oral Therapy for Erectile Dysfunction," *Sexual Medicine Reviews* 7, no. 1 (2019): 115–128.

12. Graham Jackson, H. Gillies, and I. Osterloh, "Past, Present, and Future: A 7-Year Update of Viagra (Sildenafil Citrate)," *Internal Journal of Clinical Practice* 59, no. 6 (2005): 680–691.

13. Loe, *Rise of Viagra*, 179.

14. Esther Perel, *Mating in Captivity: Reconciling the Erotic + the Domestic* (Harper-Collins, 2006), 3.

15. American Psychiatric Association, *Diagnostic and Statistical Manual of Mental Disorders*, 4th ed. (American Psychiatric Association, 2000). In 2013 this term was removed from the DSM and replaced by FSIAD, "female sexual interest/arousal disorder." Why all the fuss over nomenclature? HSDD was based on research in the 1970s that describes sexual desire as spontaneous.

16. The neuropsychopharmacologist Stephen Stahl notes that flibanserin causes increases in dopamine (DA) and norepinephrine (NE) in the brain's prefrontal cortex (PFC). DA and NE are *excitatory* with respect to sexual desire and arousal. Conversely, serotonin is *inhibitory* to sexual desire and arousal. Flibanserin also acts to decrease serotonin 5-HT (albeit transiently) in some brain areas such as the

PFC, but not others. See Stephen M. Stahl, Bernd Sommer, and Kelly A. Allers, "Multifunctional Pharmacology of Flibanserin: Possible Mechanism of Therapeutic Action in Hypoactive Sexual Desire Disorder," *Journal of Sexual Medicine* 8, no. 1 (2011): 15–27.

17. Selena McKee, "Huge Blow for Boehringer as FDA Advisors Reject Flibanserin," *PharmaTimes*, June 20, 2010, https://www.pharmatimes.com/news/huge_blow_for_boehringer_as_fda_advisors_reject_flibanserin_983051.

18. Sarah Houlton, "Female Sexual Desire Drug Approved," *Chemistry World*, August 25, 2015, https://www.chemistryworld.com/news/female-sexual-desire-drug-approved/8898.article.

19. James A. Simon, Sheryl A. Kingsberg, Brad Shumel, Vladimir Hanes, Miguel Garcia Jr., and Michael Sand, "Efficacy and Safety of Flibanserin in Postmenopausal Women with Hypoactive Sexual Desire Disorder: Results of the SNOWDROP Trial," *Menopause* 21, no. 6 (2014): 633–640.

20. Susan R. Davis, Rodney Baber, Nicholas Panay, Johannes Bitzer, Sonia Cerdas Perez, Rakibul M. Islam, et al., "Global Consensus Position Statement on the Use of Testosterone Therapy for Women," *Journal of Clinical Endocrinology and Metabolism* 104, no. 10 (2019): 4660–4666.

21. Author interview with James Simon, February 22, 2022.

22. Sheryl A. Kingsberg, Anita H. Clayton, and James G. Pfaus, "The Female Sexual Response: Current Models, Neurobiological Underpinnings and Agents Currently Approved or Under Investigation for the Treatment of Hypoactive Sexual Desire Disorder," *CNS Drugs* 29, no. 11 (2015): 915–933.

Chapter 3: Sex Today

1. Claire Groden, "Americans Sleep with Their Smartphones," *Fortune*, June 29, 2015, https://fortune.com/2015/06/29/sleep-banks-smartphones/.

2. "Study: 10 Percent of People Admit to Checking Phone During Sex," *CBS Philadelphia News*, June 7, 2018, https://www.cbsnews.com/philadelphia/news/study-10-percent-people-checking-phone-during-sex.

3. Colleen McClain and Risa Gelles-Watnick, "From Looking for Love to Swiping the Field: Online Dating in the U.S.," Pew Research Center, February 2, 2023, https://www.pewresearch.org/internet/2023/02/02/from-looking-for-love-to-swiping-the-field-online-dating-in-the-u-s/.

4. McClain and Gelles-Watnick, "From Looking for Love."

5. Abby Lee Hood and Renée Bacher, "Looking for Love? Here Are 17 Dating Apps and Websites for Over-50 Singles," AARP, January 14, 2021, https://www.aarp.org/home-family/personal-technology/info-2021/online-dating-apps.html. For example, Bumble gives women agency over the selection process—they only match with a man if they swipe on his photo and he swipes on theirs as well, and women alone can accept the match. While some are based on headshots, others hinge on personality and hobbies; some are specific to religious affiliation like Christian Mingle and

Jdate. Others, like Ourtime and Silver Singles and Datemyage are geared toward older daters. Many, including Hinge and Bumble, allow age customization. There are also LGBTQ+-friendly sites such as OkCupid, or LGBTQ+-focused ones, like Hers, Grindr, and Scruff, as well as ones specific to race or ethnicity, like BLK for the Black community or Tantan for Asian users. If you are traveling and looking for a date, it is even possible while traveling to swipe and select someone in your locale.

6. Jean M. Twenge, Ryne A. Sherman, and Brooke E. Wells, "Declines in Sexual Frequency Among American Adults, 1989–2014," *Archives of Sexual Behavior* 46, no. 8 (2017): 2389–2401.

7. Robin L. Flanigan, "The Secrets of Sex over 40: 8 Questions Answered," AARP, September 29, 2023, https://www.aarp.org/home-family/friends-family/info-2023/sex-over-40-study.html.

8. Amy Muise, Ulrich Schimmack, and Emily A. Impett, "Sexual Frequency Predicts Greater Well-Being, but More Is Not Always Better," *Social Psychological and Personality Science* 7, no. 4 (2016): 295–302.

9. Esther Perel, "Why Happy People Cheat," *The Atlantic*, October 2017, https://www.theatlantic.com/magazine/archive/2017/10/why-happy-people-cheat/537882/.

10. Jessica Klein, "Millennials in Sexless Marriages," BBC, October 20, 2022, https://www.bbc.com/worklife/article/20221019-the-millennials-in-sexless-marriages.

11. Maureen McGrath, "No Sex Marriage—Masturbation, Loneliness, Cheating and Shame," TEDxStanleyPark, July 2016, available at https://www.youtube.com/watch?v=LVgzOyHVcj4.

12. "Loneliness Is a Serious Public Health Problem," *Economist*, September 1, 2018. The *Economist* article refers to this report from the Kaiser Family Foundation: Bianca DiJulio, Liz Hamel, Cailey Muñana, and Mollyann Brodie, "Loneliness and Social Isolation in the United States, the United Kingdom, and Japan: An International Survey," Kaiser Family Foundation, August 30, 2018, https://www.kff.org/other/report/loneliness-and-social-isolation-in-the-united-states-the-united-kingdom-and-japan-an-international-survey.

13. McGrath, "No Sex Marriage."

14. Vladimir Hedrih, "The Science of Infidelity: The Key Psychological and Contextual Factors That Predict Cheating," *PsyPost*, June 25, 2024, https://www.psypost.org/the-science-of-infidelity-the-key-psychological-and-contextual-factors-that-predict-cheating.

15. Perel, "Why Happy People Cheat."

16. Elisabeth Timmermans, Elien De Caluwé, and Cassandra Alexopoulos, "Why Are You Cheating on Tinder? Exploring Users' Motives and (Dark) Personality Traits," *Computers in Human Behavior* 89 (2018): 129–139.

17. Perel, "Why Happy People Cheat."

18. "Life Expectancy by Country 2025," World Population Review, accessed August 27, 2025, https://worldpopulationreview.com/country-rankings/life-expectancy-by-country.

19. See Census.gov, at www2.census.gov/programs-surveys/demo/tables/families/time -series/marital/ms2.xls.

20. Mohit Khera, "A Simple Approach to Prolonging Your Sexspan," TEDxGreenhouse-Road, 2024, available at https://www.youtube.com/watch?v=xSe5_rh6Xk4.

21. Mohit Khera, Rajib K. Bhattacharya, Gary Blick, Harvey Kushner, Dat Nguyen, and Martin M. Miner, "The Effect of Testosterone Supplementation on Depression Symptoms in Hypogonadal Men from the Testim Registry in the US (TRiUS)," *Aging Male* 15, no. 1 (2011): 14–21.

22. Wendy Wang, "Who Cheats More? The Demographics of Infidelity in America," *Institute of Family Studies* (blog), January 10, 2018, https://ifstudies.org/blog/who -cheats-more-the-demographics-of-cheating-in-america.

23. Ethan Czuy Levine, Debby Herbenick, Omar Martinez, Tsung-Chieh Fu, and Brian Dodge, "Open Relationships, Nonconsensual Nonmonogamy, and Monogamy Among U.S. Adults: Findings from the 2012 National Survey of Sexual Health and Behavior," *Archives of Sexual Behavior* 47 (2018): 1439–1450.

Chapter 4: Desire

1. Sheryl A. Kingsberg, "Attitudinal Survey of Women Living with Low Sexual Desire," *Journal of Women's Health* 23, no. 10 (2014): 817–823.

2. The Lioness vibrator, see lioness.io.

3. Quinn, for example. I provide a list of top "audio porn" sites in an appendix at the end of this book.

4. Spontaneous desire occurs in 75 percent of men but only 15 percent of women, according to Emily Nagoski, PhD. See her website at https://www.emilynagoski .com/.

5. Emily Nagoski, *Come as You Are* (Simon & Schuster, 2015).

6. When SHBG levels are high, the body has fewer sex hormones available for use. This can lead to symptoms like low sex drive, insomnia, mood issues, vaginal dryness, and weight gain. SHBG levels can be affected by diet (flax seed increases SHBG), oral contraceptives, glucose metabolism, opioids for pain relief, medicines that affect the central nervous system, recreational drug use, eating disorders, and excessive or strenuous exercise. See F. Z. Stanczyk, Intira Sriprasert, Roksana Karim, Juliana Hwang-Levine, Wendy J. Mack, and Howard N. Hodis, "Concentrations of Endogenous Sex Steroid Hormones and SHBG in Healthy Postmenopausal Women," *Journal of Steroid Biochemistry and Molecular Biology* 223 (2022): 106080.

7. Endometriosis affects approximately 10 percent of women globally. This is about 190 million women, although its diagnosis is a rough estimate since the condition is likely underreported. See "Endometriosis," World Health Organization, March 24, 2023, https://www.who.int/news-room/fact-sheets/detail/endometriosis.

8. Gemma Sharp, Marika Tiggemann, and Julie Mattiske, "Factors That Influence the Decision to Undergo Labiaplasty: Media, Relationships, and Psychological Well-Being," *Aesthetic Surgery Journal* 36, no. 4 (2016): 469–478.

9. Wendy Macdowall, Kyle G. Jones, Clare Tanton, Soazig Clifton, Andrew J. Copas, Catherine H. Mercer, et al., "Associations Between Source of Information About Sex and Sexual Health Outcomes in Britain: Findings from the Third National Survey of Sexual Attitudes and Lifestyles (Natsal-3)," *BMJ Open* 5, no. 3 (2015): e007837.

10. Annika L. Rasmussen, Søren V. Larsen, Brice Ozenne, Kristin Köhler-Forsberg, Dea S. Stenbæ, Martin B. Jørgensen, et al., "Sexual Health and Serotonin 4 Receptor Brain Binding in Unmedicated Patients with Depression—a NeuroPharm Study," *Transnational Psychiatry* 13 (2023).

11. Amy Muise, Ulrich Schimmack, and Emily A. Impett, "Sexual Frequency Predicts Greater Well-Being, but More Is Not Always Better," *Social Psychological and Personality Science* 7, no. 4 (2016): 295–302; Edward Laumann, Anthony Paik, Dale B. Glasser, Jeong-Han Kang, Tianfu Wang, Bernard Levinson, et al., "A Cross-National Study of Subjective Sexual Well-Being Among Older Women and Men: Findings from the Global Study of Sexual Attitudes and Behaviors," *Archives of Sexual Behavior* 35 (2006): 145–161.

12. Lisa Dawn Hamilton and Cindy M. Meston, "Chronic Stress and Sexual Function in Women," *Journal of Sexual Medicine* 10, no. 10 (2013): 2443–2454.

13. To see what I mean in a coffee table book version of what could be titled *The United Colors of Vulva*, check out the GynoDiversity Project, https://gynodiversity.com/.

14. Emily Morse, *Smart Sex* (HarperCollins, 2023), 117.

15. Imago Relationships: https://imagorelationships.org/.

Chapter 5: Pleasure

1. Emily Morse, *Smart Sex* (HarperCollins, 2023), 13.

2. The number of truly asexual humans is not easy to quantify but estimates range from 1 to 2 percent.

3. *Nag* is an oft-used word I detest. "I nag well and often and am proud to be called a nag, a nagging nag, a hag who nags," said no woman ever.

4. Kate Manne, *Entitled: How Male Privilege Hurts Women* (Crown, 2020), 11.

5. Morse, *Smart Sex*, 62.

6. Laura Hawks, Steffie Woolhandler, David U. Himmelstein, David H. Bor, Adam Gaffney, and Danny McCormick, "Association Between Forced Sexual Initiation and Health Outcomes Among US Women," *JAMA Internal Medicine* 179, no. 11 (2019): 1551–1558.

7. https://www.aasect.org is the website for the American Association of Sexuality Educators, Counselors, and Therapists, and it is an easy way to locate a professional for sex therapy or to get certified as a sex therapist.

8. Mark Travers, "A Psychologist Explains the Long-Term Effects of Your First Sexual Experience," *Forbes*, May 27, 2024, https://www.forbes.com/sites/traversmark/2024/05/27/a-psychologist-explains-the-long-term-effects-of-your-first-sexual-experience/.

9.   The biological anthropologist Helen Fischer studied the nature of love and why one human is attracted to another. Her book *Anatomy of Love* is a must-read if you want to nerd out on why you love who you love, and the history of mating and courtship. It is also a comprehensive look at the social sexual world we live in now. Fischer became the chief science officer at Match.com; she also created a scale by which people may be characterized by neurochemical types and social behaviors. Every human, she believed, was a unique mixture of one of four types: the Explorers, creative and curious with high levels of dopamine; Builders, conscientious rule followers with high serotonin levels; Directors, characterized by high testosterone levels, aggressive and competitive, yet logical; and Negotiators, who seek consensus and are nurturing, with high estrogen levels. What type are you? And what type are you attracted to?

10. Helen E. Fisher, Arthur Aron, and Lucy L. Brown, "Romantic Love: A Mammalian Brain System for Mate Choice," *Philosophical Transactions of the Royal Society B: Biological Sciences* 29, no. 361 (2006): 2173–2186.

11. J. Thomas Curtis, Yan Liu, Brandon J. Aragona, and Zuoxin Wang, "Dopamine and Monogamy," *Brain Research* 1126 (2006): 76–90.

12. A. H. Clayton et al., "Bupropion as an Antidote to SSRI-Induced Sexual Dysfunction," poster presented at the New Clinical Drug Evaluation Unit Program (NCDEU), Boca Raton, FL, May 30, 2000–June 2, 2000.

13. Anita H. Clayton, James F. Pradko, Harry A. Croft, C. Brendan Montano, Robert A. Leadbetter, Carolyn Bolden-Watson, et al., "Prevalence of Sexual Dysfunction Among Newer Antidepressants," *Journal of Clinical Psychiatry* 63 (2002): 357–366.

14. M. S. Exton, T. H. Krüger, M. Koch, E. Paulson, W. Knapp, U. Hartmann, et al., "Coitus-Induced Orgasm Stimulates Prolactin Secretion in Healthy Subjects," *Psychoneuroendocrinology* 26, no. 3 (2001): 287–294.

15. S. Brody and T. H. Krüger, "The Post-Orgasmic Prolactin Increase Following Intercourse Is Greater Than Following Masturbation and Suggests Greater Satiety," *Biological Psychology* 71, no. 3 (2006): 312–315.

Chapter 6: The Orgasm Gap

1.   Lara Eschler, "The Physiology of the Female Orgasm as a Proximate Mechanism," *Sexualities, Evolution & Gender* 6, nos. 2/3 (2004): 171–194.

2.   Elizabeth A. Armstrong, Paula England, and A. C. K. Fogarty, "Orgasm in College Hookups and Relationships," in *Families as They Really Are*, ed. B. J. Risman (W. W. Norton, 2009).

3.   David A. Frederick, H. Kate St. John, Justin R. Garcia, and Elizabeth A. Lloyd, "Differences in Orgasm Frequency Among Gay, Lesbian, Bisexual, and Heterosexual Men and Women in a U.S. National Sample," *Archives of Sexual Behavior* 47 (2018): 273–288.

4.   "Facial": a directorial favorite, in which semen is ejaculated onto the face of the "willing" recipient.

5. Lux Alptraum, *Faking It: The Lies Women Tell About Sex—and the Truths They Reveal* (Seal Press, 2018), 48.

6. M. J. E. Klaassen and Jochen Peter, "Gender (In)equality in Internet Pornography: A Content Analysis of Popular Pornographic Internet Videos," *Journal of Sex Research* 52, no. 7 (2015): 721–735.

7. Léa J. Séguin, Carl Rodrigue, and Julie Lavigne, "Consuming Ecstasy: Representations of Male and Female Orgasm in Mainstream Pornography," *Journal of Sex Research* 55 (2018): 348–356.

8. Talia Shirazi, Kaytlin J. Renfo, Elisabeth Lloyd, and Kim Wallen, "Women's Experience of Orgasm During Intercourse: Question Semantics Affect Women's Reports and Men's Estimates of Orgasm Occurrence," *Archives of Sexual Behavior* 47, no. 3 (2018): 605–613.

9. Anna Moore and Coco Khan, "The Fatal, Hateful Rise of Choking During Sex," *Guardian*, July 25, 2019, https://www.theguardian.com/society/2019/jul/25/fatal-hateful-rise-of-choking-during-sex.

10. Devon J. Hensel, Christiana D. von Hippel, Charles C. Lapage, and Robert H. Perkins, "Women's Techniques for Making Vaginal Penetration More Pleasurable: Results from a Nationally Representative Study of Adult Women in the United States," *PLoS One* 16, no. 4 (2021): e0249242.

11. Debby Herbenick, Heather Eastman-Mueller, Tsung-Chieh Fu, Brian Dodge, Kia Ponander, and Stephanie A. Sanders, "Women's Sexual Satisfaction, Communication, and Reasons for (No Longer) Faking Orgasm: Findings from a U.S. Probability Sample," *Archives of Sexual Behavior* 48, no. 8 (2019): 2461–2472.

12. Herbenick, Eastman-Mueller, Fu, Dodge, Ponander, and Sanders, "Women's Sexual Satisfaction."

13. Author interview with Christine Claypoole, December 2024.

14. Kelly Casperson, *You Are Not Broken: Stop Should-ing All over Your Sex Life* (Sheldon Press, 2024), 95.

15. G. Davey Smith, S. Frankel, and J. Yarnell, "Sex and Death: Are They Related? Findings from the Caerphilly Cohort Study," *British Medical Journal* 315, no. 7123 (1997): 1641–1644.

16. I suggest patients use 2 percent topical testosterone cream applied nightly to the clitoris for six weeks and then once weekly thereafter.

17. With thanks to Kelly Casperson for that perfect analogy.

18. Alptraum, *Faking It*, 24 and 12.

Chapter 7: The Five *M*'s

1. Kabat-Zinn developed MBSR in 1979 when he treated patients with chronic illness using meditation; his techniques are now used in over seven hundred hospitals worldwide. See "Jon Kabat-Zinn: Defining Mindfulness," Mindful.org, January 11, 2017, https://www.mindful.org/jon-kabat-zinn-defining-mindfulness/.

2. Jon Kabat-Zinn, "Opening Meditation: Mindfulness in the Modern Age," San Francisco, 2024, YouTube video, https://www.youtube.com/watch?v=tLRw9IQFFRk; and Kabat-Zinn, "Opening Meditation," Mindfulness in America Summit, New York, 2018, available at https://www.youtube.com/watch?v=5zGTORjxyTc.

3. Resources for locating CBT therapists can be found at services.abct.org; references for hypnosis therapy can be found at asch.net; for sex therapists at aasect.org; for mindfulness-based stress reduction at goodtherapy.org or the MasterClass with Jon Kabat-Zinn.

4. Robert E. Pyke, "Sexual Performance Anxiety," *Sexual Medicine Reviews* 8, no. 2 (2020): 183–190.

5. "Family Planning/Contraception Methods," World Health Organization, https://www.who.int/news-room/fact-sheets/detail/family-planning-contraception.

6. To find a pelvic floor physical therapist, use the PT locator on the website of the academy of the American Physical Therapy Association: https://www.aptapelvichealth.org/ptlocator.

7. Leah J. Elias, Isabella K. Succi, Melanie D. Schaffler, William Foster, Mark A. Gradwell, Manon Bohic, et al., "Touch Neurons Underlying Dopaminergic Pleasurable Touch and Sexual Receptivity," *Cell* 186, no. 3 (2023): 577–590.

8. Ian Sample, "Origins of Masturbation Traced Back to Primates 40m Years Ago," *Guardian*, June 6, 2023, https://www.theguardian.com/science/2023/jun/07/origins-masturbation-traced-back-primates-40m-years-ago#.

9. Thomas Szasz, *The Second Sin* (Anchor Press, 1973), 10.

10. Emily Nagoski, *Come as You Are*, 2nd ed. (Simon and Schuster, 2021), 319.

11. Jan L. Shifren, Brigitta U. Monz, Patricia A. Russo, Anthony Segreti, and Catherine B. Johannes, "Sexual Problems and Distress in United States Women: Prevalence and Correlates," *Obstetrics and Gynecology* 112 (2008): 970–978; Gabriela S. Pachano Pesantez and Anita H. Clayton, "Treatment of Hypoactive Sexual Desire Disorder Among Women: General Considerations and Pharmacological Options," *Focus* 19, no. 1 (2021): 39–45. The definition of HSDD was modified by the International Society for the Study of Women's Sexual Health in 2018 to include the duration of symptoms and distress. See Anita H. Clayton, Irwin Goldstein, Noel N. Kim, Stanley E. Althof, Stephanie S. Faubion, Brooke M. Faught, et al., "The International Society for the Study of Women's Sexual Health Process of Care for Management of Hypoactive Sexual Desire Disorder in Women," *Mayo Clinic Proceedings* 93 (2018): 467–487.

12. Anita H. Clayton, Evan R. Goldfischer, Irwin Goldstein, Leonard Derogatis, Diane J. Lewis-D'Agostino, and Robert Pyke, "Validation of the Decreased Sexual Desire Screener (DSDS): A Brief Diagnostic Instrument for Generalized Acquired Female Hypoactive Sexual Desire Disorder (HSDD)," *Journal of Sexual Medicine* 6, no. 3 (2009): 730–738.

13. James G. Pfaus, Amama Sadiq, Carl Spana, and Anita H. Clayton, "The Neurobiology of Bremelanotide for the Treatment of Hypoactive Sexual Desire Disorder in Premenopausal Women," *CNS Spectrums* 27, no. 3 (2022): 281–289.

14. Susan R. Davis, Rodney Baber, Nicholas Panay, Johannes Bitzer, Sonia Cerdas Perez, Rakibul M. Islam, et al., "Global Consensus Position Statement on the Use of Testosterone Therapy for Women," *Climacteric* 22, no. 5 (2019): 429–434.
15. Conversation with Kelly Casperson, May 3, 2025.
16. T. van Staa and J. Sprafka, "Study of Adverse Outcomes in Women Using Testosterone Therapy," *Maturitas* 62 (2009): 76–80.
17. Abdulmaged M. Traish and Louis J. Gooren, "Safety of Physiological Testosterone Therapy in Women: Lessons from Female-to-Male Transsexuals (FMT) Treated with Pharmacological Testosterone Therapy," *Journal of Sexual Medicine* 7 (2010): 3758–3764.

Chapter 8: Repositioning Sex Ed

1. Jamie Kravitz, "Naomi Watts Gets Candid About Menopause, Owning Her Story and Self-Care," *Good Housekeeping*, June 25, 2024, www.goodhousekeeping.com/life/entertainment/a64341391/naomi-watts-stripes-beauty-menopause-interview/.
2. "Naomi Watts on How Peri-Menopause Personally Inspired Her Pro-Aging Beauty Brand," Breakfast Television, YouTube video, accessed August 27, 2025, https://www.youtube.com/watch?v=y7pWI3w2x0k.
3. "Shredding the Silence on Menopause with Tamsen Fadal," *Hot Flashes and Cool Topics* podcast, October 23, 2024, available at https://open.spotify.com/episode/6ZWIVVsF8571KxqpUQj7Jw.
4. The fertile window for most women is from around five days before ovulation through the day after ovulation.
5. "roofied": refers to sexual encounter, usually nonconsensual, after being given Rohypnol or other drugs. See "The Teen Trend of Sex Choking," *New York Times*, April 4, 2025, https://www.nytimes.com/2024/04/25/opinion/teen-sex-choking.html.
6. "Mean Girls," Paramount, accessed August 27, 2025, https://www.paramountpictures.com/movies/mean-girls.
7. "Demystifying Data Tool Kit," Guttmacher Institute, accessed August 27, 2025, https://www.guttmacher.org/sites/default/files/report_downloads/demystifying-data-handouts_0.pdf.
8. "Sex Education and HIV Education," Guttmacher Institute, accessed July 17, 2025, https://www.guttmacher.org/state-policy/explore/sex-and-hiv-education.
9. Anna Katz, "Sex Ed Goes Global: The Netherlands," Duke University, Center for Global Reproductive Health, July 19, 2018, https://dukecenterforglobalreproductivehealth.org/2018/07/19/sex-ed-goes-global-the-netherlands/.
10. Bonnie J. Rough, "How the Dutch Do Sex Ed," *The Atlantic*, August 29, 2018, www.theatlantic.com/family/archive/2018/08/the-benefits-of-starting-sex-ed-at-age-4/568225/.
11. Philp M. Sarrel, David Portman, Patrick Lefebvre, Marie-Hélène Lafeuille, Amanda Melina Grittner, Jonathan Fortier, et al., "Incremental Direct and Indirect Costs of Untreated Vasomotor Symptoms," *Menopause* 22, no. 3 (2015): 260–266.

12. "NASEM Releases Report Assessing Women's Health Research at NIH," Society for Women's Health Research, December 6, 2024, https://swhr.org/nasem-releases-report-assessing-womens-health-research-at-nih.

13. "Appendix B, Key Trends in Demographic Diversity in Clinical Trials," in *Improving Representation in Clinical Trials and Research: Building Research Equity for Women and Underrepresented Groups*, ed. Kirsten Bibbins-Domingo and Alex Helman (National Academies Press, 2022), available at https://www.ncbi.nlm.nih.gov/books/NBK584392.

14. Lin Yang and Adetunji T. Toriola, "Menopausal Hormone Therapy Use Among Postmenopausal Women," *JAMA Health Forum* 5, no. 9 (2024): e243128.

15. Philip M. Sarrel, Valentine Y. Njike, Valentina Vivante, and David L. Katz, "The Mortality Toll of Estrogen Avoidance: An Analysis of Excess Deaths Among Hysterectomized Women Aged 50 to 59 Years," *American Journal of Public Health* 103, no. 9 (2013): 1583–1588.

16. I love words! Here is a cool one: *fornication*. The Italian word for ant is *formica* (plural *formiche*), so you can see where we get formication, the sensation of ants crawling on your skin. From interview with Wen Shen, November 4, 2024.

17. Author interview with Wen Chen, November 4, 2024.

18. Mindy S. Christianson, Jennifer A. Ducie, Kristiina Altman, Ayatalla M. Khafagy, and Wen Shen, "Menopause Education: Needs Assessment of American Obstetrics and Gynecology Residents," *Menopause* 20, no. 11 (2013): 1120–1125.

19. Juliana M. Kling, Kathy L. MacLaughlin, Peter F. Schnatz, Carolyn J. Crandall, Lisa J. Skinner, Cynthia A. Stuenkel, et al., "Menopause Management Knowledge in Postgraduate Family Medicine, Internal Medicine and Obstetrics and Gynecology Residents: A Cross-Sectional Survey," *Mayo Clinic Proceedings* 94, no. 2 (2019): 242–253.

20. The market research firm Grand View Research valued the global menopause market at $17.79 billion in 2024 and projects it will grow to $24.35 billion by 2030. PreScouter projects the menopause market to reach $600 billion by 2030, citing the huge economic potential in the femtech industry and that currently only 7 percent of femtech startups focus on menopause-related solutions.

21. Hui Lui, Linda Waite, Shannon Shen, and Donna Wang, "Is Sex Good for Your Health? A National Study on Partnered Sexuality and Cardiovascular Risk Among Older Men and Women," *Journal of Health and Social Behavior* 57, no. 3 (2016): 276–296.

22. Shannon Criniti, Betsy Crane, Mark B. Woodland, Owen C. Montgomery, and Sandra Urdaneta Hartmann, "Perceptions of U.S. Medical Residents Regarding Amount and Usefulness of Sexual Health Instruction in Preparation for Clinical Practice," *American Journal of Sexuality Education* 11, no. 3 (2016): 161–175.

23. Ilona Plug, Sandra van Dulmen, Wyke Stommel, Tim C. Olde Hartman, and Enny Das, "Physicians' and Patients' Interruptions in Clinical Practice: A Quantitative Analysis," *Annals of Family Medicine* 20, no. 5 (2002): 423–429; Kari A. Phillips,

Naykky Singh Ospina, and Victor M. Montori, "Physicians Interrupting Patients," *Journal of General Internal Medicine* 34, no. 10 (2019): 1965.

24. Plug, van Dulmen, Stommel, Hartman, and Das, "Physicians' and Patients' Interruptions in Clinical Practice."
25. "Femtech Market: Global Forecast (2025–2034)," Global Market Insights, accessed July 17, 2025, gminsights.com/industry-analysis/femtech-market/amp.

Chapter 9: Toys, Lube, Erotica, and Virtual Reality

1. Antonia Vallentin, *Picasso* (Cassell, 1963), 168.
2. Timothy Clark, *Shunga: Sex and Pleasure in Japanese Art* (Brill, 2013).
3. Maria Ahlin, "Let's Talk Porn," TedxGöteborg, February 2019, available at https://www.youtube.com/watch?v=DBTb71UzPmY.
4. Erika Lust, "The Porn Conversation," TedxAthens, May 2022, available at https://www.youtube.com/watch?v=PnK9Y7yuGWg.
5. Sara Dobie Bauer, Louisa Ballhaus, and Alice Kelly, "27 Erotic Sex Scene Excerpts from Books That Leave You Begging for More," She Knows, March 20, 2025, https://www.sheknows.com/feature/hottest-sex-scenes-romance-novels-1838224/.
6. Information from LELO.com.
7. "Avoid Toxic Chemicals," Women's Voices for the Earth, accessed July 17, 2025, https://womensvoices.org/avoid-toxic-chemicals/.
8. Joelle M. Brown, Kristen L. Hess, Stephen Brown, Colleen Murphy, Ava Lena Waldman, and Marjan Hezareh, "Intravaginal Practices and Risk of Bacterial Vaginosis and Candidiasis Infection Among a Cohort of Women in the United States," *Obstetrics and Gynecology* 121, no. 4 (2013): 773–780.
9. "Sex Toys Market Size, Share and Trends Analysis Report by Product (Vibrators, Masturbation Sleeves, Dildos, Sex Dolls), by Distribution Channel (E-Commerce, Specialty Stores), by Region, and Segment Forecasts, 2024–2030," Grand View Research, https://www.grandviewresearch.com/industry-analysis/sex-toys-market.
10. Another word to know is *teledildonics* (or *cyberdildonics*). Wikipedia defines this as virtual sex encounters using networked electronic sex toys to mimic and extend human sexual interaction (https://en.wiktionary.org/wiki/teledildonics). The *Collins Dictionary* definition is one of a technology supposedly enabling two or more people to engage in sexual activity remotely (https://www.collinsdictionary.com/us/dictionary/english/teledildonics#google_vignette).
11. Sonia Milani, Faith Jabs, Natalie B. Brown, Bozena Zdaniuk, Alan Kingstone, and Lori A. Brotto, "Virtual Reality Erotica: Exploring General Presence, Sexual Presence, Sexual Arousal, and Sexual Desire in Women," *Archives of Sexual Behavior* 51, no. 1 (2022): 565–576.
12. This detects the six degrees of freedom in space (up/down, left/right, forward/backward) in which the pose of the wearer is being tracked.
13. "VR Porn Industry Statistics," Bedbible Research Center, accessed July 17, 2025, https://bedbible.com/vr-porn-industry-statistics/.

Chapter 10: Other Bedroom Gaps

1. David A. Frederick, Brian Joseph Gillespie, Janet Lever, Vincent Berardi, and Justin R. Garcia, "Debunking Lesbian Bed Death: Using Coarsened Exact Matching to Compare Sexual Practices and Satisfaction of Lesbian and Heterosexual Women," *Archives of Sexual Behavior* 50, no. 8 (2021): 3601–3619.

2. Nicholas C. Bene, Peter C. Ferrin, Jing Xu, Geolani W. Dy, Daniel Dugi III, and Blair R. Peters, "Tissue Options for Construction of the Neovaginal Canal in Gender-Affirming Vaginoplasty," *Journal of Clinical Medicine* 8, no. 13 (2024): 2760.

3. And remember, these medications aren't safe for everyone, including men with cardiovascular disease and elevated blood pressure. Talk with your doctor to be sure you are a candidate.

4. Joan Price, *Naked at Our Age* (Seal Press, 2011), 199.

5. Price, *Naked at Our Age*, 206–207.

6. "Diabetes," Center for Disease Control, accessed July 17, 2025, https://www.cdc .gov/diabetes.

7. "Relationships and Sex After a Heart Attack," Heart Foundation, accessed July 17, 2025, https://www.heartfoundation.org.au/your-heart/support/relationships-sex-after -a-heart-attack.

8. Sonali Shah, "'Disabled People Are Sexual Citizens Too': Supporting Sexual Identity, Well-Being, and Safety for Disabled Young People," *Frontiers in Education* 2 (2017), full text at https://www.frontiersin.org/journals/education/articles/10.3389/feduc .2017.00046/full.

9. "Disability and Health Overview," Center for Disease Control and Prevention, April 2, 2025, https://www.cdc.gov/disability-and-health/about/.

10. Tom Shakespeare, Kath Gillespie-Sells, and Dominic Davies, *The Sexual Politics of Disability: Untold Desires* (Cassell, 1996).

11. Elizabeth Holdsworth, Viktoriya Trifonova, Clare Tanton, Hannah Kuper, Jessica Datta, Wendy Macdowall, et al., "Sexual Behaviors and Sexual Health Outcomes Among Young Adults with Limiting Disabilities: Findings from Third British National Survey of Sexual Attitudes and Lifestyles (Natsal-3)," *BMJ Open* 8, no. 7 (2018): e019219.

12. "Mission and History," Chronic Sex, accessed July 17, 2025, https://www.chronicsex .org/mission-history/.

13. Maria Grazia Maggio, Patrizia Calatozzo, Antonio Cerasa, Giovanni Pioggia, Angelo Quartarone, and Rocco Salvatore Calabrò, "Sex and Sexuality in Autism Spectrum Disorders: A Scoping Review on a Neglected but Fundamental Issue," *Brain Science* 12, no. 11 (2022): 1427.

14. In 1900 the global average life expectancy was thirty-two years, forty-seven years in the United States. By 2021 it had more than doubled to seventy-one years globally, seventy-nine years in the United States. See "Social Explorer Analysis for New York Times Finds 80-Year-Olds Aren't Limited to White House," *Social*

Explorer (blog), November 22, 2022, https://www.socialexplorer.com/blog/post
/social-explorer-analysis-for-new-york-times-finds-80-year-olds-arent-limited-to
-white-house-13049.

15. "Fact Sheet: Aging in the United States," Population Reference Bureau, accessed
August 28, 2025, https://www.prb.org/resources/fact-sheet-aging-in-the-united
-states/.

16. Katherine Schaeffer, "U.S. Centenarian Population Is Projected to Quadruple over
the Next 30 Years," Pew Research Center, January 9, 2024, https://www.pewresearch
.org/short-reads/2024/01/09/us-centenarian-population-is-projected-to-quadruple
-over-the-next-30-years/.

17. "Let's Talk About Sex," National Poll on Healthy Aging, University of Michigan, May
2018, https://deepblue.lib.umich.edu/bitstream/handle/2027.42/143212/NPHA
-Sexual-Health-Report_050118_final.pdf.

18. "Let's Talk About Sex." Side note: When a patient sixty to eighty years old asked a
doctor about a sexual problem, the conversation was initiated by the doctor less than
half the time.

19. "Fact Sheet: Aging in the United States."

20. Betty Dodson, "Introduction," in Price, *Naked at Our Age*, 3–4.

Appendix One: Sex Positions for People with Disabilities

1. "Sex Positions for Disabilities, a Comprehensive Guide," Ro, accessed August 28,
2025, https://ro.co/health-guide/sex-positions-for-disabilities/.

Appendix Two: Podcasts, Porn Sites, Oh My

1. Anna Borges, "Audio Porn Is Helping Women Connect with Their Sexuality on
Their Terms: Here's 17 Places to Tune In and Turn On," *Glamour*, April 11, 2024,
https://www.glamourmagazine.co.uk/article/audio-porn-erotica.

Index

About the Author

Maria Sophocles, MD, FACOG, MSCP, IF, is an internationally renowned gynecologist and thought leader in menopause and female sexual function. A longtime advocate for women's health, she fought to pass legislation to secure access to contraception in New Jersey in 2023, pioneered the use of carbon dioxide lasers on the vulva and in the vagina to regenerate unhealthy tissue, and started a women's clinic in rural Kenya. A frequent commentator on Sirius XM's *Doctor Radio* and TED speaker, Maria lives in Princeton, New Jersey, where she heads a progressive gynecological clinic that serves over 30,000 women.